Disclaimer: This textbook is not intended to provide, and disclaims any suggestion that it does provide, medical advice of any nature. The information made available through this textbook should not be used in place of seeking professional opinions by licensed practitioners. Only licensed medical professionals may offer medical advice, diagnosis and recommendations for treatment of medical conditions. You assume full responsibility for appropriate use of the information available through this textbook.

As Medicine is an ever-changing science, with new research and clinical experience, changes in treatment and techniques are required. The authors have checked with sources believed to be reliable in effort to provide information that is complete and generally in accord with standards accepted at the time of publication. The opinions expressed in this work represent those of the authors and, in view of the possibility of human error or changes in medical science, neither the authors, RAEducation.com LLC, nor any other party who has been involved in the preparation or publication of this work warrants that the information contained herein is in every respect accurate or complete and they are not responsible for any errors or omissions or for the results obtained from the use of such information. Readers and viewers are encouraged to confirm the information contained herein with other sources.

Published by RAEducation.com LLC Publications, Gainesville, FL USA
Produced by Kristine Lyle, Printers Workshop, Kalona, IA

ISBN-10: 1-948083-11-6
ISBN-13: 978-1-948083-11-9

André P. Boezaart
MBChB, MPraxMed, DA(CMSA), FFA(CMSA), MMed(Anesth), PhD
Professor of Anesthesiology and Orthopaedic Surgery
Division of Acute and Peri-operative Pain Medicine
Acute Pain Service
University of Florida College of Medicine, Gainesville, Florida, USA

Cameron R. Smith
M.D., Ph.D.
Assistant Professor of Anesthesiology
Division of Acute and Peri-operative Pain Medicine
Acute Pain Service
University of Florida College of Medicine, Gainesville, Florida, USA

Johan P. Reyneke
B.Ch.D., M.Ch.D., FCFMOS(SA), Ph.D.
Director, Centre for Orthognathic Surgery,
Cape Town Mediclinic, Cape Town, South Africa
Honorary Professor, Department of Maxillofacial & Oral Surgery
University of the Western Cape, Cape Town, South Africa
Associate Professor, Division of Oral and Maxillofacial Surgery
Universidad Autonoma de Nuevo Leon, Monterrey, Mexico
Clinical Professor, Department of Oral & Maxillofacial Surgery
University of Oklahoma College of Dentistry, Oklahoma City, Oklahoma, USA
Clinical Professor, Department of Oral and Maxillofacial Surgery
University of Florida College of Dentistry, Gainesville, Florida, USA

Artwork by:
Mary K. Bryson, MAMS, CMI
Bryson Biomedical Illustration
Langhorne, Pennsylvania

Educational electronic and printed media for the website
RAEducation.com owned by RAEducation.com LLC.

Please visit www.RAEducation.com
for video tutorials on this and other topics

The Pterygopalatine Ganglion Block

Introduction

The pterygopalatine ganglion (PPG), often described as the "Piccadilly Circus of the Face," is of great importance to anesthesiologists, pain physicians, neurologists and surgeons, and its blockade is becoming more and more popular as our understanding of the cholinergic mechanisms of headache improve.[1] It is also known as the sphenopalatine ganglion, Meckel's ganglion or the Nasal ganglion. Recent publications have shed important light on the neuroanatomy and neurophysiology of this ganglion and its relationship with the trigeminal ganglion, and, more important, its role in the pathophysiology of vascular or primary headaches. This, and the applied macroanatomy, sonoanatomy, surface anatomy and microanatomy of this ganglion will be discussed in much detail in this book, as well as popular techniques of performing the pterygopalatine ganglion block.

Indications for PPG Block

Not only is the pterygopalatine ganglion block (PPGB) becoming more widely used and popular for post-operative pain management for surgeries, such as cleft palate, maxillary osteotomy, maxillectomy in cancer surgery, functional endoscopic sinus surgery and tonsillectomy, it is also starting to show very promising results for primary headaches, which include acute and chronic migraine, tension-type headache, and trigeminal autonomic cephalgias, which include cluster headache and postdural puncture headache.

Currently, apart from diagnostic blocks to assist with the diagnosis and management of many chronic pain conditions of musculoskeletal, vascular and neurogenic origin, it is obviously highly indicated and effective for acute and perioperative pain situations for surgeries in the territory of the maxillary nerve and its branches (See section on Applied Anatomy). Accepted indications for PPGB include: persistent idiopathic facial pain,[2] pterygo-palatine (Sluder's neuralgia)[3] and trigeminal neuralgia (tic douloureux),[4] herpes zoster involving the ophthalmic nerve, and a variety of other facial neuralgia.[5,6] Other emerging indications for PPGB include musculoskeletal pain, especially of the head, neck, shoulders and back[6,7,8] and complex regional pain syndrome.[8] Ruskin promoted the PPGB for the treatment of myofascial pain originating from the trapezius and sternocleidomastoid muscles in 1959. Since then other researchers have used it successfully for myofascial pain and fibromyalgia.[10] Pain resulting from head and neck cancer can be severe and difficult to manage. In certain patients, trans nasal PPGB can be effectively self-administered at home to manage chronic pain.[11]

The Pathophysiology of Primary Headaches

Classification of Headache

Part 1: The Primary Headaches			
1	Migraine	1. 2.	Acute Chronic
2	Tension-Type Headache		
3	Trigeminal Autonomic Headaches	1. 2. 3.	Cluster Headache Paroxysmal Hemicrania Hemicrania Continua
4	Other Primary Headache Disorders	1. 2. 3. 4.	Postdural Puncture Headache Stimulus-induced Headache Thunderclap headache New Daily Persistent Headache
Part 2: Secondary Headaches			
	Headaches or Facial Pain Attributed to:	1. 2. 3. 4. 5. 6. 7. 8. 9. 10.	Trauma to Head and/or Neck Cranial or Cervical Vascular Disease Neurovascular Intracranial Disorder Substance or its Withdrawal Infection Disorder of Homeostasis Disorder of Cranium, Neck, Eyes, Ears, Nose, Sinuses, Teeth, Mouth, or Other Facial or Cervical Structures Psychiatric Disorders Giant Cell Arthritis Medication Overuse Headache
Part 3: Painful Cranial Neuropathies			
	Painful Cranial Neuropathies, Other Facial Pain, and Other Headaches	1. 2.	Painful cranial neuropathies Other headache disorders

Table 1: The International Classification of Headache Disorders

The International Classification of Headache Disorders (ICHD) was first published in 1988 and has now gone through 2 revisions, most recently in 2013. The classification is freely available online at https://www.ichd-3.org.

Basic Anatomic Principles
Somatic and Autonomic Connections and Their Origins

The PPG, a complex neural center with multiple connections to trigeminal, fascial and autonomic systems, consists of somatosensory, sympathomotor and parasympathetic fibers. The sensory distribution is to the nose, throat, hard and soft palates and paranasal sinuses and orbit. It probably derives its motor root from the nervus intermedius (glossopatatinus or Wrisberg nerve) through the greater petrosal nerve and may consist of parasympathetic efferent (preganglionic) fibers from the medulla. The PPG motor fibers form synapses with neurons whose postganglionic axons are distributed with the deep branches of the trigeminal nerve. These postganglionic axons are parasympathetic and form the secreto-motor innervation of the mucous membranes of the nose, soft palate, tonsils, uvula, roof of the mouth, upper lip, gums and the upper part of the pharynx.[1,2,3]

The PPG autonomic innervation is complex and extremely important in understanding the rationale of the PPGB for primary headaches. The PPG sympathetic root is derived from the internal carotid plexus from the superior cervical ganglion and passes via the deep petrosal nerve to the PPG. The greater superficial petrosal nerve and the deep petrosal nerve join to form the nerve of the pterygoid canal (Vidian nerve) before entering the PPG. (See Fig. 1)

The PPG parasympathetic root has its preganglionic origin in the superior salivary nucleus in the medulla oblongata. These fibers pass through the nervus intermedius, the facial nerve, the geniculate ganglion, and the greater petrosal nerve to reach the PPG via the Vidian nerve in the pterygoid canal (Fig 1).

The greater superficial petrosal nerve also carries taste fibers along with the presynaptic parasympathetic fibers to the soft palate via the lesser palatine nerve, while the parasympathetic fibers synapse in the PPG and postsynaptic fibers supply secretomotor function to the lacrimal gland, mucosa of the palate, nasopharynx and nasal cavity. All of this functional anatomy is essential to allow us to understand the effects and side effects of blocking these functions of the PPG.

Although the peripheral effects and side effects are easy to explain and understand (anesthesia and analgesia) how does this all relate to primary headache? Overall, the PPG is important for intraocular pressure balance and cerebral vasodilatation associated with vascular originated headaches.[13] Recent research has highlighted the important role of the PPG in cerebrovascular autonomic physiology, in the pathophysiology of cluster and migraine headaches, and in conditions such as stroke and cerebral vasospasm.[14] Let us expand on this.

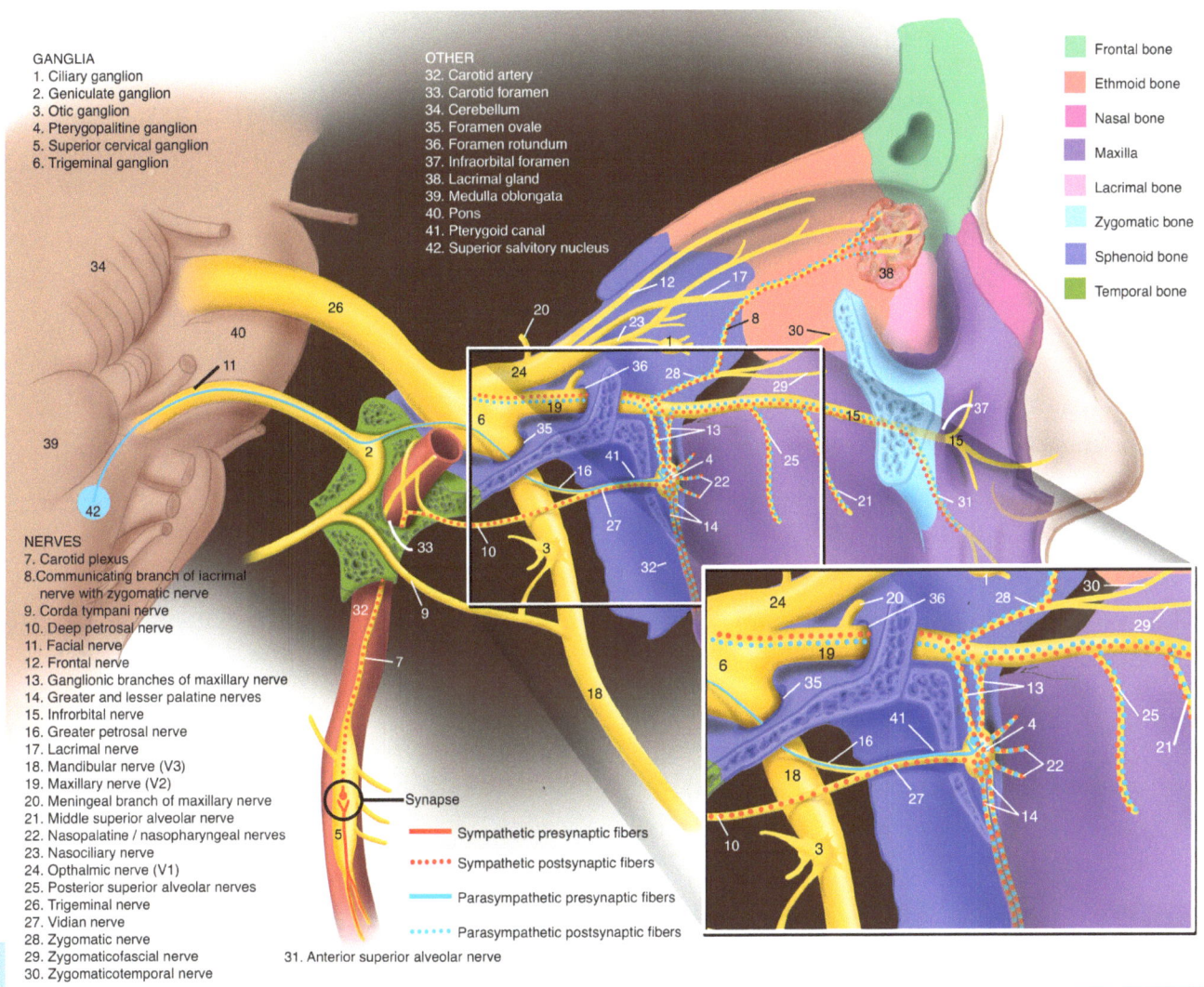

GANGLIA
1. Ciliary ganglion
2. Geniculate ganglion
3. Otic ganglion
4. Pterygopalitine ganglion
5. Superior cervical ganglion
6. Trigeminal ganglion

OTHER
32. Carotid artery
33. Carotid foramen
34. Cerebellum
35. Foramen ovale
36. Foramen rotundum
37. Infraorbital foramen
38. Lacrimal gland
39. Medulla oblongata
40. Pons
41. Pterygoid canal
42. Superior salvitory nucleus

Frontal bone
Ethmoid bone
Nasal bone
Maxilla
Lacrimal bone
Zygomatic bone
Sphenoid bone
Temporal bone

NERVES
7. Carotid plexus
8. Communicating branch of lacrimal nerve with zygomatic nerve
9. Corda tympani nerve
10. Deep petrosal nerve
11. Facial nerve
12. Frontal nerve
13. Ganglionic branches of maxillary nerve
14. Greater and lesser palatine nerves
15. Infrorbital nerve
16. Greater petrosal nerve
17. Lacrimal nerve
18. Mandibular nerve (V3)
19. Maxillary nerve (V2)
20. Meningeal branch of maxillary nerve
21. Middle superior alveolar nerve
22. Nasopalatine / nasopharyngeal nerves
23. Nasociliary nerve
24. Opthalmic nerve (V1)
25. Posterior superior alveolar nerves
26. Trigeminal nerve
27. Vidian nerve
28. Zygomatic nerve
29. Zygomaticofascial nerve
30. Zygomaticotemporal nerve

31. Anterior superior alveolar nerve

Synapse

—— Sympathetic presynaptic fibers
••••• Sympathetic postsynaptic fibers
—— Parasympathetic presynaptic fibers
••••• Parasympathetic postsynaptic fibers

11

Figure 1: Schematic depiction of the afferent and efferent sympathetic and parasympathetic innervation of the pterygopalatine ganglion.

Recent microanatomical studies[15] of the PPG revealed a neural 'scaffold' with trigeminovascular projections and trigeminal-autonomic plexus. (See Fig. 13 in Microanatomy Section). Within the PPG, and on the posterior wall of the maxillary sinus, distinctive trigeminovascular projections were demonstrated. Rusu[15] concluded that the evidence that he presented of a microscopic parasympathetic "bridging" neural network between the PPG and the tri- geminal ganglion via the pterygopalatine trigeminovascular scaffold – anastomotic trigeminal branches, offers a substrate for better understanding of various facial algias and cephalgias. This study of Rusu gave evidence that sustains the existence of an anatomically defined pterygopalatine-trigeminovascular system (PPTVS).

This is important, because blood vessels of the brain, pia mater and dura mater are innervated by a dense network of unmyelinated nerve fibers. For all the supratentorial structures, the innervation originates from the trigeminal ganglion, constituting the trigeminovascular system (TVS); whereas for the subtentorial structures, the innervation originates from the dorsal root of the upper cervical roots,[16] which are now known to be connected by this scaffold of microanatomical anastomoses.[15] This network is mainly parasympathetic and is responsible for vasodilatation.

According to modern concepts, the general key step of pathogenesis of various craniofacial pain syndromes, including primary headaches (tension-type headache, migraine, cluster headache and postdural puncture headache (PDPH)) is activation of the trigeminal nerve, which is followed by the formation of an ascending nociceptive flow along the trigemino-thalamo-cortical pathway.[17-19] The trigeminal nerve is the main source of sensory innervation of the head tissue, which form the functional trigeminovascular system (TVS) together with the intracranial vessels. This system is very important in the pathophysiology of primary cephalgias. The branches of the facial (greater petrosal nerve) and glossopharyngeal (lesser petrosal nerve) nerves provide parasympathetic innervation of the intracranial structures. Blocking the PPG, will therefore counter the vasodilatory effect on the cerebral, pial and dural vessels.

New data and clinical observations conclusively show that trigeminal neurons, which receive meningeal nociceptive stimuli trigger parasympathetic flow. This parasympathetic flow in turn, initiates and maintains development of aseptic meningeal vasculitis, which additionally activates and/or sensitizes the meningeal nociceptors.[20] Due to the formation of this vicious circle, parasympathetic transmission grows progressively and this results not only in aggravation of the current attack, but also chronization of the headache. The breaking of this vicious circle may significantly alleviate a patient's condition. Data on the efficiency of various therapeutic interventions at the pterygopalatine ganglion level, specifically blocking with local anesthetics and corticosteroids,[21-22] radio frequency ablation,[23] neurostimulation[24] and onabotuliniumtoxin A (Botox) injection[25] at the PPG, for alleviating and preventing cluster headache, migraine, and PDPH, strongly support this conclusion.

Acetylcholine, as well as other parasympathetic neurotransmitters, may be considered as a vasoactive substance and a modulator of nociception. Acetylcholine is an important independent regulator of intracranial circulation. It mostly exerts a vasodilator effect on the wall of the cranial arteries, which allows us to consider acetylcholine as a potential pain-provoking agent in all types of vascular headaches. Intracranial and extracranial vasodilatation is considered as epiphenomenon of primary neuronal impairment in the pathogenesis of cephalgias.[1]

Why would Botox injection on the PPG be effective, since it is believed not to have effects on nerves? Recent data of two pilot studies[25,26] demonstrated that Botox injection around the PPG were followed by a significant decrease in the number of days with moderate and severe headache in patients with chronic migraine and chronic cluster headache.[25] It has been suggested that Botox can, via axonal transport, reach the central terminals of the trigeminal nociceptors[26] and exert a central anti-nociceptive effect, probably due to involvement of the opioidergic system.[26]

Migraine, Cluster Headache & Postdural Puncture Headache

Migraine attack develops due to trigeminovascular activity,[27] which is induced spontaneously or after the action of some exoxogenous and/or endogenous factor under the condition of insufficient inborn or acquired activity of the descending anti-nociceptive system.[28-32] This results in the development of aseptic neurogenic inflammation of meningeal vessels, due to antidromic release of various vasoactive factors, including calcitonin gene-related peptide (CGRP), neurokinin A, nitric oxide, glutamine and substance P from the terminals of the trigeminal afferents. Under conditions of meningo-vasculitis, orthodromic stimulation of A-delta-fibers and C-fibers of the trigeminal nerve occurs. These transmit nociceptive information from the cerebral and meningeal vessels to the spinal nucleus, where primary sensory processing takes place. The information then goes to the upper structures of the central nervous system.[33] Neurovascular impairments together with growing nociceptive traffic are followed by sensitization of peripheral and central parts of the trigemino-thalamo-cortical pathway, which is expressed as the specific pain syndrome, cutaneous allodynia, and accompanying autonomic symptoms.

Migraine Pathophysiology can thus be viewed upon a background of a presumably genetically induced hypersensitivity of the brain to both internal and external homeostatic changes that can act as triggers. These triggers influence the trigeminovascular system (TVS), which contain both peripheral and central nervous system components. Stimulation of the TVS results in the release of neuropeptides and other substances that cause both local inflammation and distal amplification of neural circuitry in the brain-stem, trigeminal nucleus caudalis, thalamus, and cortex, leading to central sensitization and symptom worsening along with reduced activity in central descending inhibitory systems and reduced ability to control or extinguish the headache attack.[34]

Strong parasympathetic activity and dysfunction of the hypothalamus play a leading role in the pathogenesis of **Cluster Headache**. This determines the classical clinical picture, including fascicular severe pain with a specific circadian rhythm, associated tearing, rhinorrhea, myosis, ptosis and periorbital edema on the affected side.[6,35] An increase in the parasympathetic tone in dilatation of intracranial vessels, their higher permeability, development of edema of the vascular wall, and finally, stimulation of the perivascular trigeminal afferents, which, in turn, close the loop of the trigeminal-facial reflex with respective progressive pathologic enhancement of the autonomic mediation.[33] The impairment of the hypothalamic control disinhibits the trigeminovascular traffic at the level of the spinal nucleus, and probably determines the clear rhythmicity of pain attacks.

Not much is known about the pathophysiology of **Postdural Puncture Headache**, but clear evidence exists of cerebral vasodilatation following accidental dural puncture.[36] Furthermore, known cerebral vascular constrictors such as caffeine and theophylline – and the most powerful of them all, peridural hematoma (epidural blood patch), relieve the headache. There is no reason to believe that the pathogenesis of all three these conditions is not the same, although caused by different factors. The treatment of all three is the same: pterygopalatine ganglion block.

Anatomy of the Pterygopalatine Ganglion

1	Pterygomaxillary fissure -----	6	Sphenoid bone
2	Pterygopalatine fossa - - - -	7	Pterygoid bone
3	Inferior orbital fissure	8	Zygomatic process
4	Maxilla	9	Temporal bone
5	Pterygoid plate	→	Pterygopalatine canal

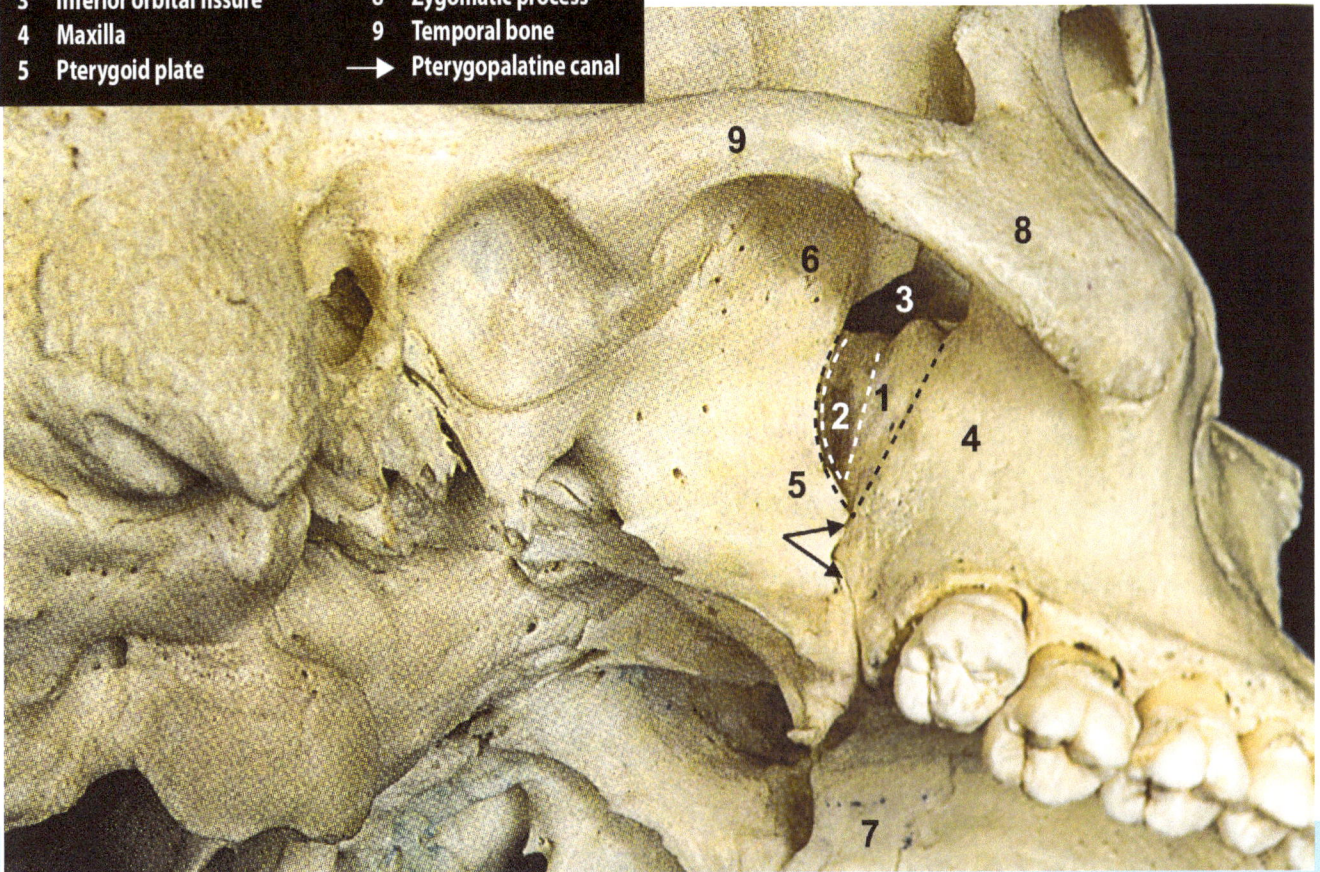

Figure 2: The pterygopalatine fossa.

Applied Macroanatomy

The pterygomaxillary fissure (1) is a triangular space between the inferotemporal or posterior aspect of the maxilla (4), which contains the maxillary sinus and the pterygopalatine plate (5). The pterygopalatine fossa (2) is more medial between the pterygoid plate (5) posterior and the palatine bone anteromedial. Superiorly, the fissure is situated anterior to the infratemporal surface of the greater wing of the sphenoid bone (6). At its superior wider base is the inferior orbital fissure (3). At the inferior apex of the triangular space, the pterygopalatine canal is found (indicated by the arrows). This pterygomaxillary fissure leads into the pterygopalatine fossa, which houses the pterygopalatine ganglion. Figure 2 also shows the pterygoid bone (7), the zygomatic process (8) and the zygomatic process of the temporal bone (9).

Perhaps these images explain the relationships between the facial bones better.

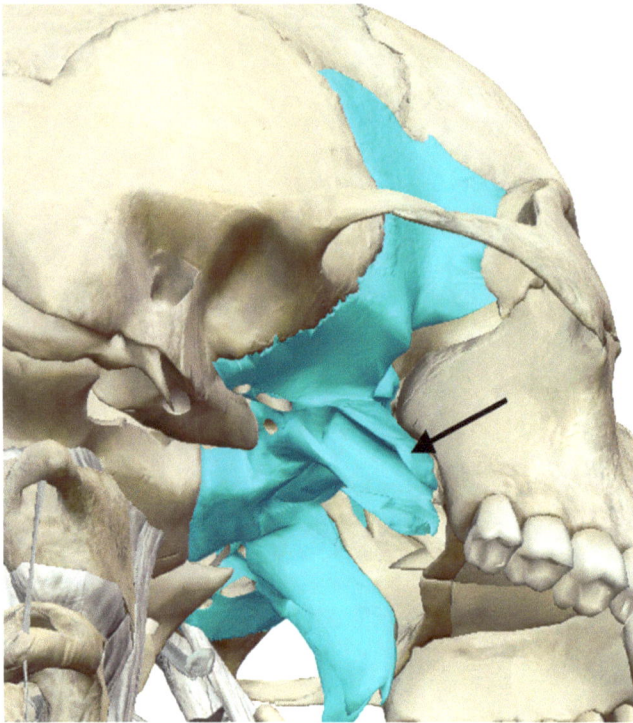

Figure 3A: The sphenoid bone (blue) with the arrow indicating the lateral pterygoid plate.

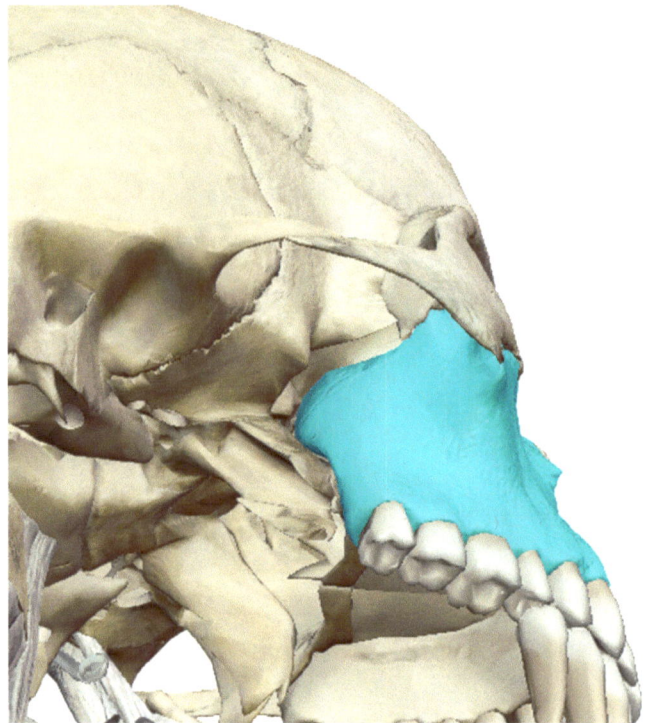

Figure 3B: The maxilla (blue)

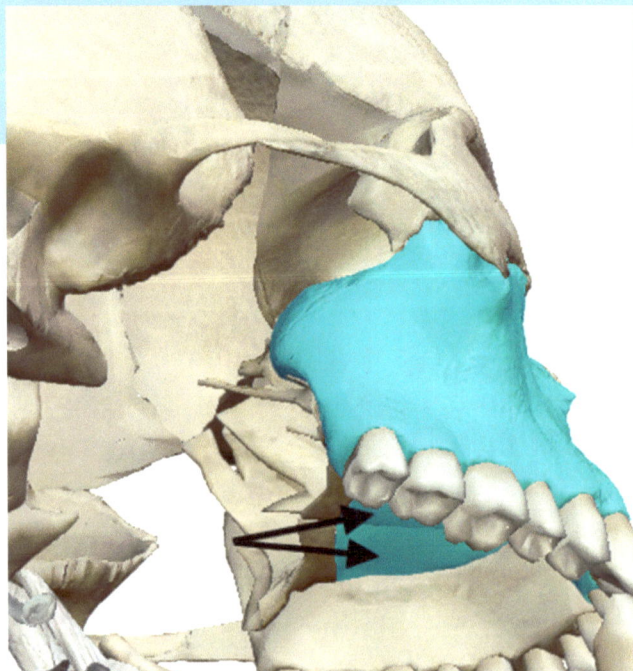

Figure 3C: The maxilla (blue) with the two bones of the hard palate (arrows).

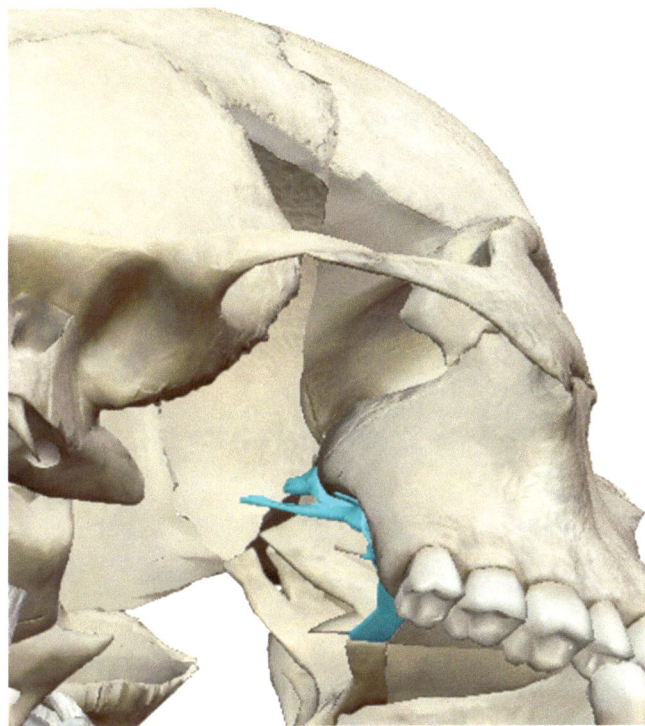

Figure 3D: The pterygoid bone (blue). (Sphenoid bone removed).

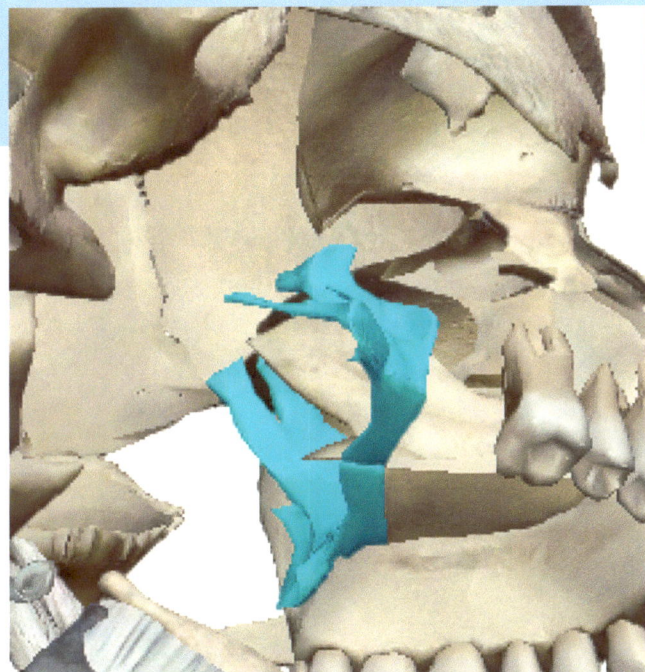

Figure 3E:The palatine bone (blue). (Maxilla and ethmoid bones removed)

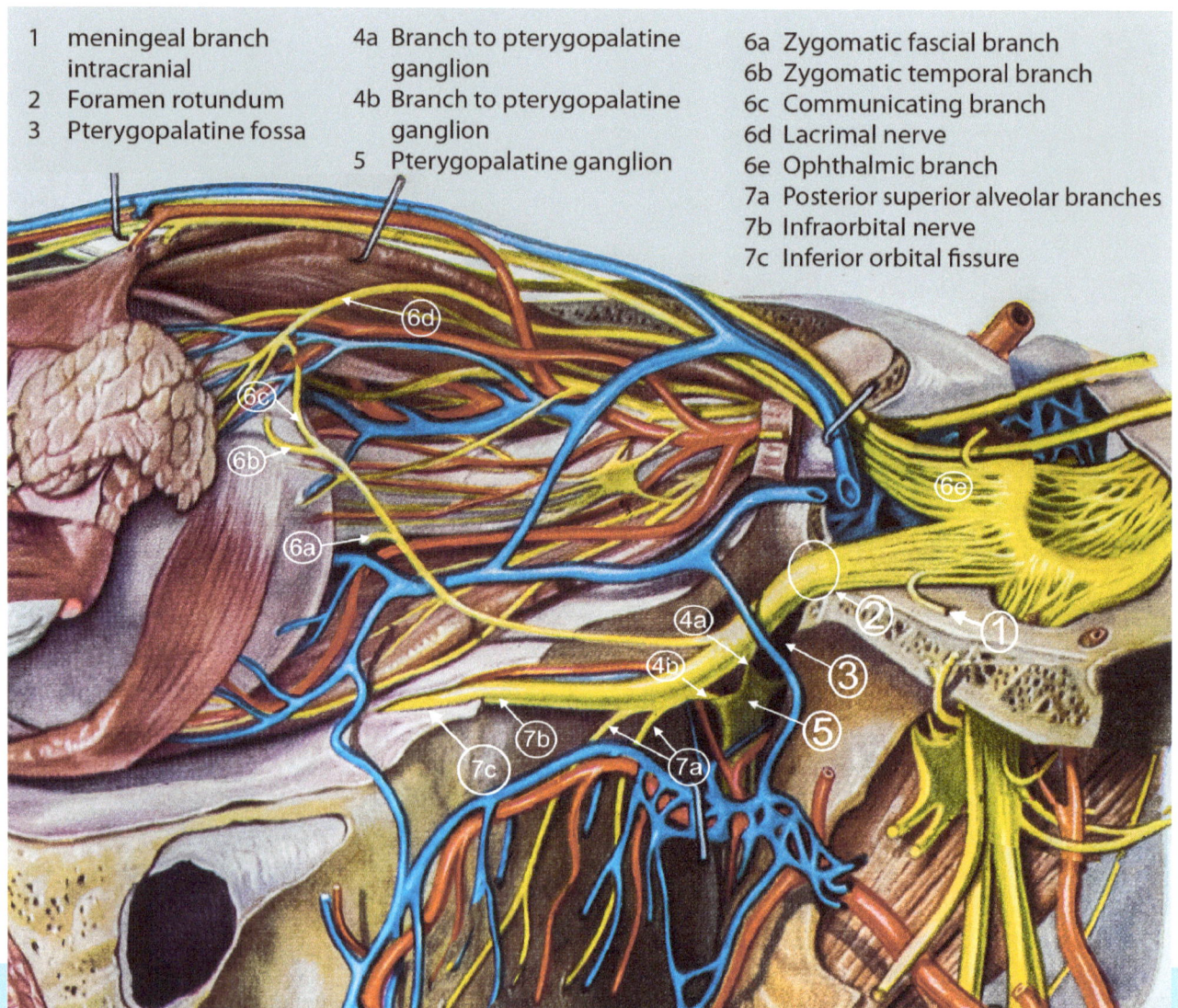

1 meningeal branch intracranial
2 Foramen rotundum
3 Pterygopalatine fossa
4a Branch to pterygopalatine ganglion
4b Branch to pterygopalatine ganglion
5 Pterygopalatine ganglion
6a Zygomatic fascial branch
6b Zygomatic temporal branch
6c Communicating branch
6d Lacrimal nerve
6e Ophthalmic branch
7a Posterior superior alveolar branches
7b Infraorbital nerve
7c Inferior orbital fissure

18

Figure 4: Lateral view of the orbit, middle cranial fossa and the pterygopalatine fissure illustrating the direct branches of the maxillary nerve.

The illustration above (Figure 4) identifies the maxillary nerve, or the middle branch (2nd division) of the trigeminal nerve (Vth cranial nerve) or trigeminal (Gasserian) ganglion. While still intracranial, the maxillary nerve gives off the 1st of its six branches: The dural or meningeal branch (1). It then passes through the foramen rotundum (2) to enter the pterygopalatine fossa (3) near the inferior orbital fissure, which connects the pterygopalatine fossa with the orbit.

Here it gives off two branches (4a and 4b) to the pterygopalatine ganglion (5), which is also called the sphenopalatine ganglion, Meckel's ganglion or the nasal ganglion.

It continues further anterior in the pterygopalatine fossa and gives of a zygomatic branch, which then enters the orbit and splits into three branches:

1. Zygomatic facial branch (6a)
2. Zygomatic temporal branch (6b) and
3. A communicating branch (6c) to the lacrimal branch (6d) of the ophthalmic nerve (6e). This communicating branch is a parasympathetic secretomotor nerve that originates from the pterygo-palatine ganglion.

Further anterior, still in the pterygopalatine fossa, the maxillary nerve gives off one or two posterior superior alveolar branches, which innervates the three upper molar teeth. The maxillary nerve then continues further anterior as the infra-orbital nerve (7b).

The infra-orbital nerve (7b) enters the orbit through the inferior orbital fissure (7c) and runs anterior in the infra-orbital groove in the floor of the orbit where it gives off the middle superior alveolar branch that innervate the premolar teeth. It then enters the infra-orbital canal to exit from the inferior orbital foramen just inferior to the infra-orbital ridge. Here the infra-orbital nerve splits into three terminal branches, the inferior palpebral branch that innervates the lower eyelid, the nasal branch and the superior labral branch.

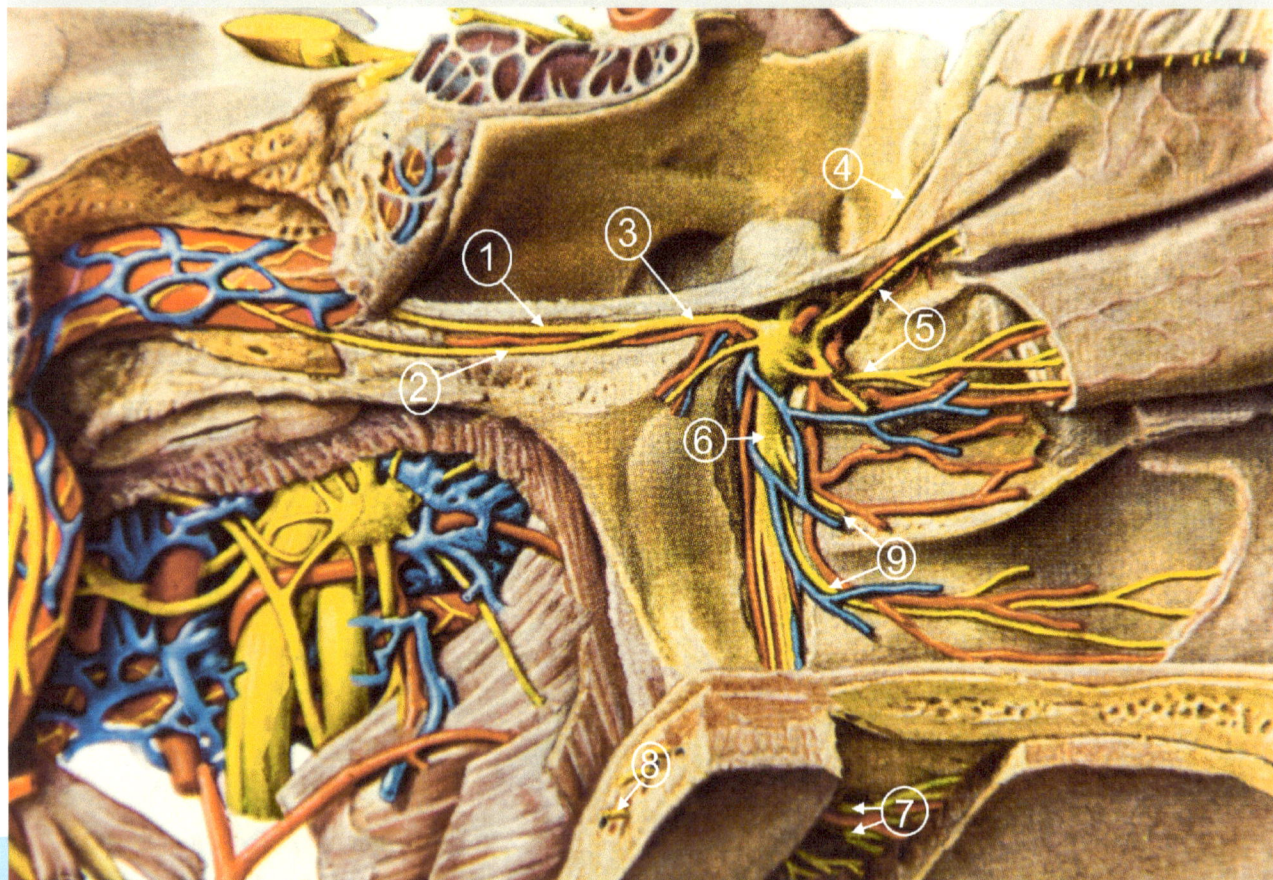

1 greater petrosal nerve
2 deep petrosal nerve
3 Vidian nerve
4 orbital branches
5 nasal branches
6 palatine nerve
7 branches of the greater palatine nerve
8 branches of the lesser palatine nerve
9 nasal branches of the palatine nerve

Figure 5: Lateral view of pterygopalatine ganglion depicting autonomic branches to the ganglion (1, 2 & 3) and indirect branches of the maxillary nerve (4 – 9)

The pterygopalatine ganglion not only receives sensory fibers from the maxillary nerve, it also receives preganglionic parasympathetic fibers from the superior salivatory nucleus in the medulla oblongata. These fibers pass, via the geniculum of the facial nerve, to become the greater petrosal nerve (1). The greater petrosal nerve then enters the pterygopalatine canal where it joins the deep petrosal nerve (2), a purely sympathetic nerve, to form the Vidian nerve (3).

The preganglionic parasympathetic nerves form synapses in the pterygopalatine ganglion and the postganglionic parasympathetic nerves are secretomotor. The sympathetic nerves originate from the superior cervical ganglion, and are thus postganglionic nerves that pass with the internal carotid artery and are vasomotor nerves.

All the indirect maxillary nerve branches (the branches that go through the ganglion (4-9)) are postganglionic and contain sympathetic vasomotor fibers, parasympathetic secretomotor fibers, and somatic touch, pain and temperature fibers.

The maxillary nerve has six indirect branches that go through the pterygopalatine ganglion of which five pick up sympathetic and parasympathetic fibers on their way through it. These are:

1. Orbital branches (4) that innervate the orbital periosteum, and the sphenoidal sinus mucosa.
2. Posterior superior nasal branches (5), which splits into medial and lateral branches. One of the medial (septal) branches continue to enter through the anterior incisive fossa of the palate as the nasopalatine nerve.
3. Palatine nerve (6), which courses inferiorly through the pterygopalatine canal where it splits into the greater, anteri-

or (7) and lesser, posterior branches (8) of the nerve. The lesser palatine nerve innervates the soft palate and the tonsils. The greater palatine nerve innervates the hard palate, and also gives off at least 2 nasal branches (9) on its way through the pterygopalatine canal.

Interestingly, taste fibers that originate from the solitary nucleus in the lower medulla oblongata, tract via the facial nerve, and split off to join the great petrosal nerve, the Vidian nerve and the lesser palatine nerve and supply it with taste fibers – hence, taste buds in the soft palate.

All the direct and indirect branches of the maxillary nerve are blocked with a pterygopalatine block.

Applied Sonoanatomy

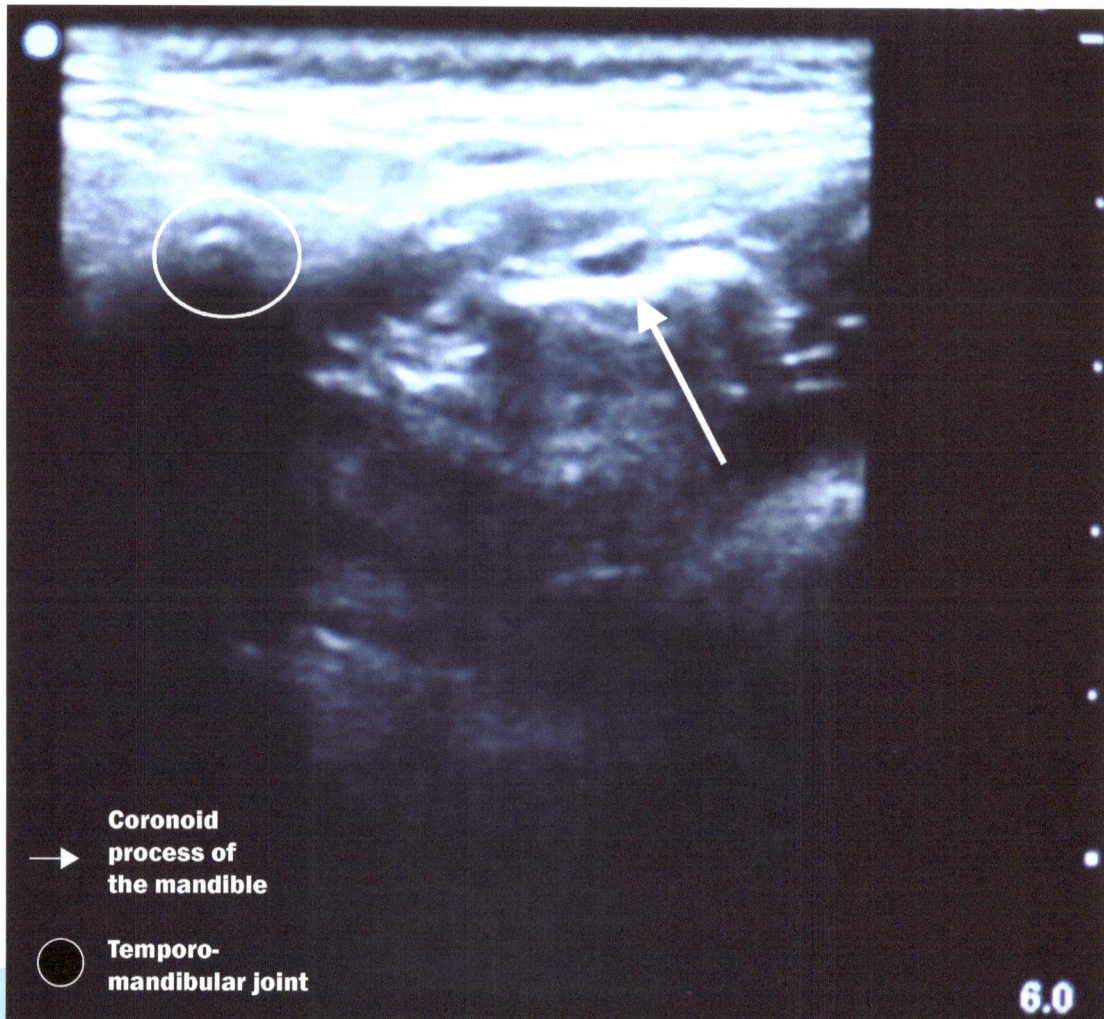

Coronoid process of the mandible

Temporo-mandibular joint

6.0

Figure 6: Ultrasound picture shows the temporo-mandibular joint (white circle) and coronoid process of the mandible (white arrow).

Identify specifically the temporo-mandibular joint (white circle) and the coronoid process (arrow) of the mandible.

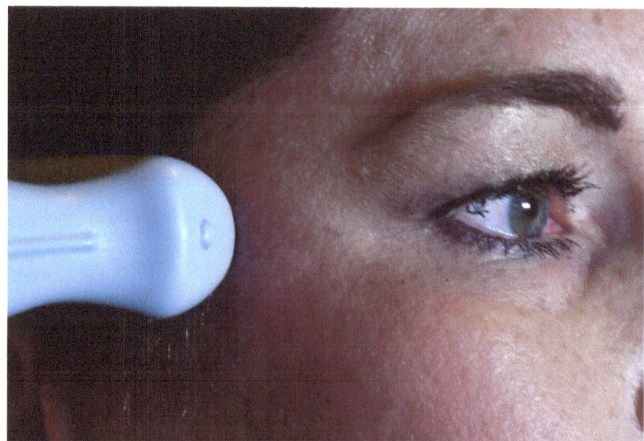

Figure 7: Lateral view of the right side of the face: The ultrasound probe is placed on the posterior aspect of the frontal process of the zygomatic bone.

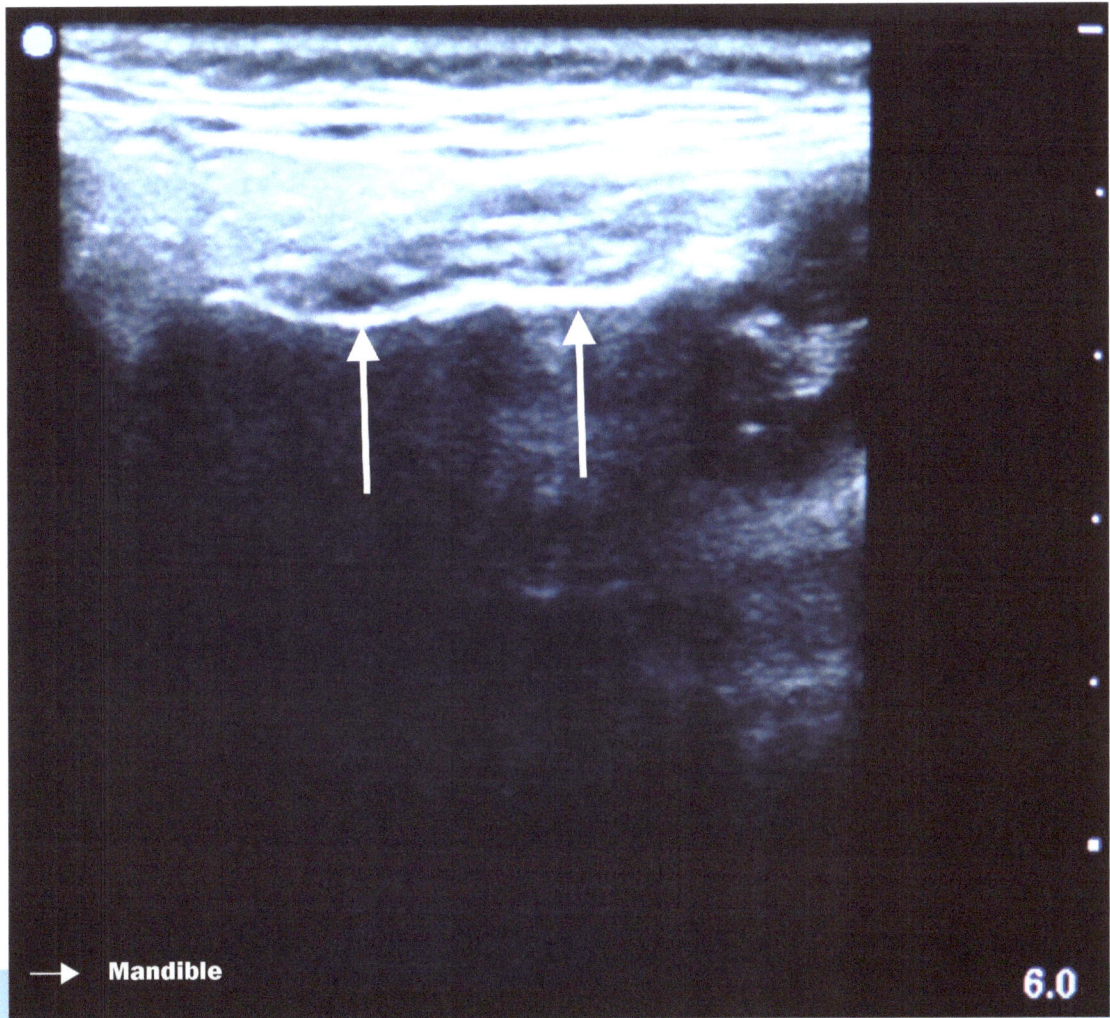

Mandible

6.0

Figure 8: When the probe is moved caudally, the coronoid notch will disappear and the mandible will appear as one flat structure (white arrows).

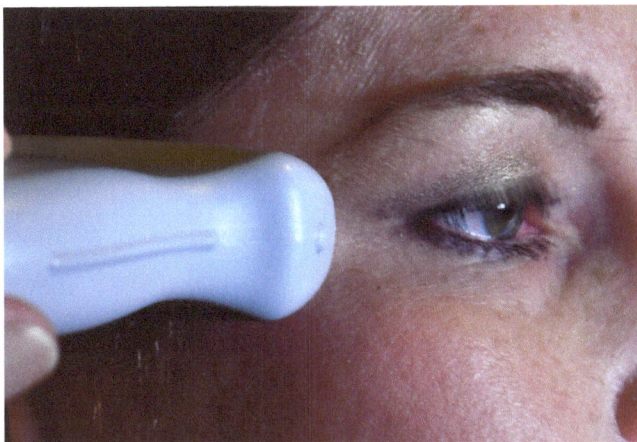

Figure 9: A lateral view of the right side of the face: Moving the probe anteriorly on the zygomatic bone.

The ultrasound probe is now placed more anteriorly on the zygomatic arch (Fig. 9). As the ultrasound probe is moved further caudally, the coronoid process should join the condylar process just past the mandibular notch (Arrows in Fig. 8). The coronoid notch disappears and the mandible becomes one flat bony structure.

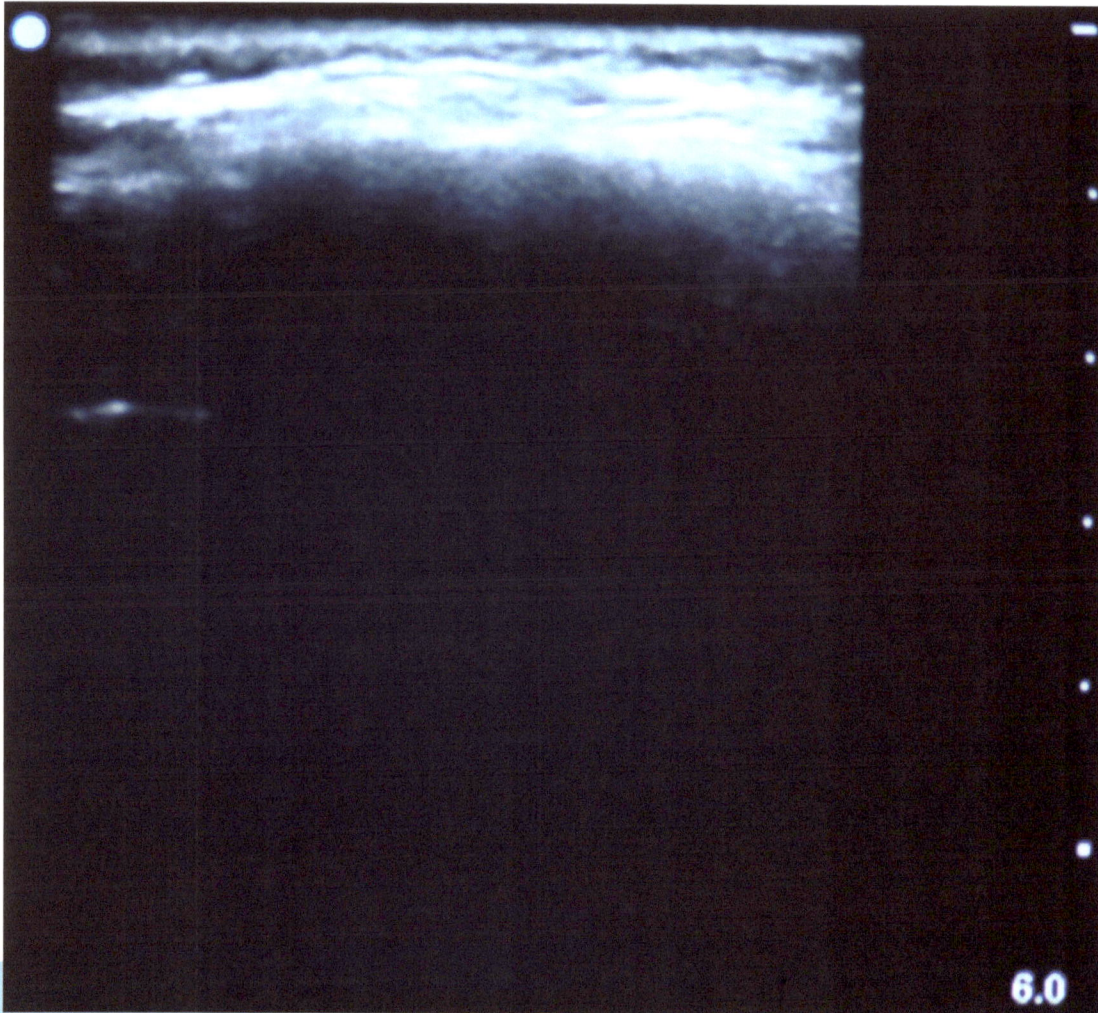

6.0

Figure 10: By moving the probe anteriorly, the sonogram shows the zygomatic bone.

The ultrasound probe is now moved caudally, 'slipping off' the zygomatic bone (Fig. 11). This picture depicts the zygomatic arch as seen on the ultrasound screen (Fig. 10).

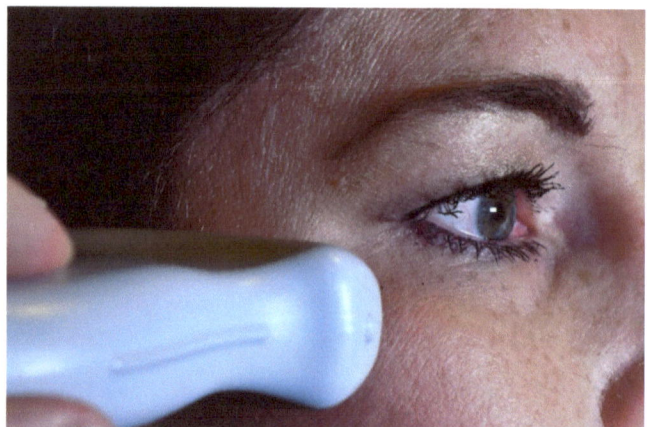

Figure 11: A lateral view of the right side of the face: Slip the ultrasound probe off the zygoma.

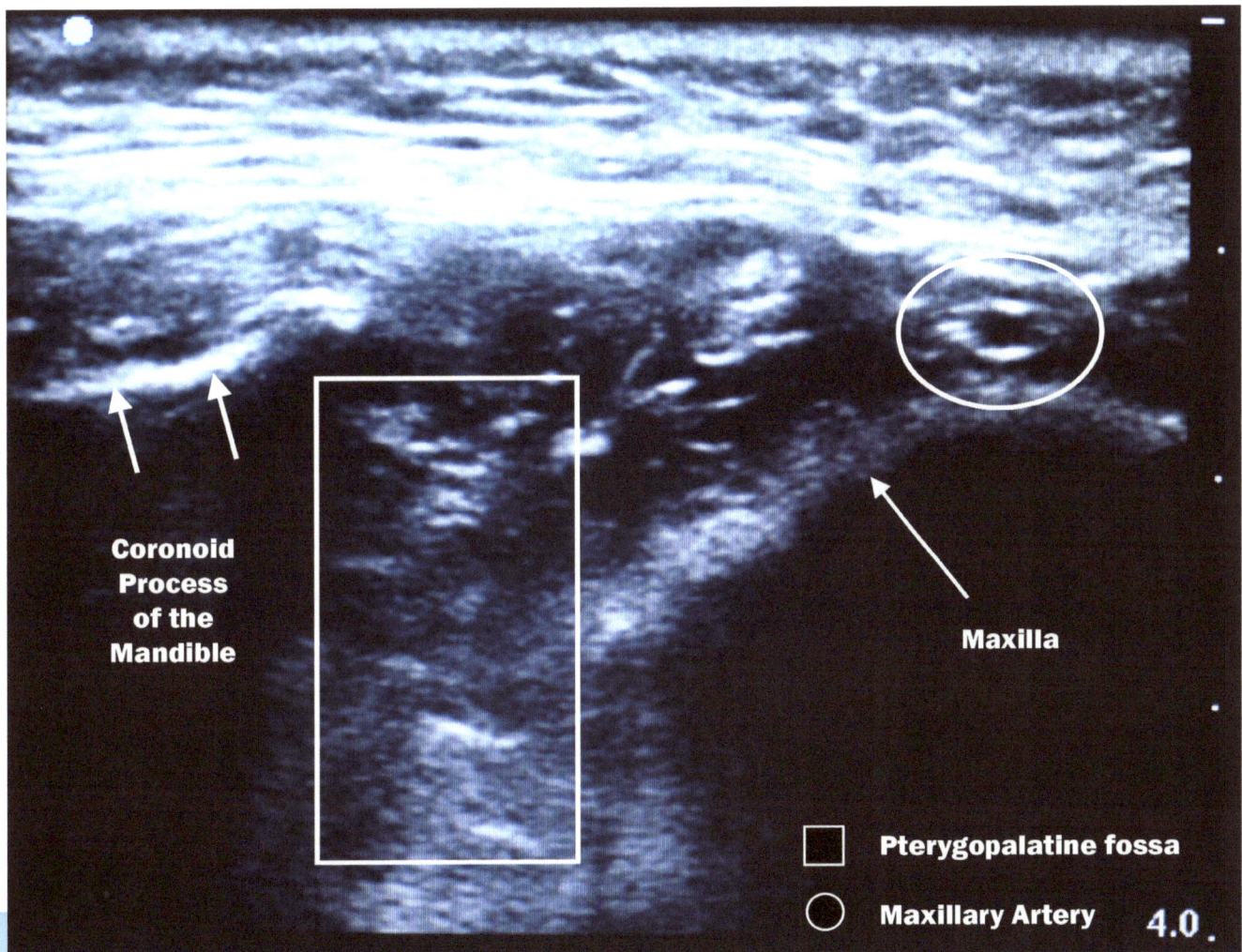

Coronoid Process of the Mandible

Maxilla

☐ **Pterygopalatine fossa**

○ **Maxillary Artery** 4.0

Figure 12: Pterygopalatine fossa with its content (white restangle), the maxilla (single arrow) and coronoid process of the mandible (double arrows).

Moving the probe caudad shows the pterygopalatine fossa with its content (white rectangle), the maxilla (white arrow) and the coronoid process of the mandible (double white arrows). When the mouth is opened the coronoid process moves out of the field and the greater wing of the sphenoid bone comes into view. The pterygopalatine fossa, which houses the pterygopalatine ganglion is indicated by the rectangle.

Note the arch formed by the maxilla on the right-hand side (single arrow). Also note the branch of the maxillary artery (circle), which can be seen pulsating.

The coronoid process of the mandible (double arrows) and, sometimes, in babies and preadolescents, the cartilaginous infra-temporal surface of the greater wing of the sphenoid bone allows the sphenoid sinus to be visible. This is almost never possible in older children or adults, due to the relative thickness of the same infra-temporal surface (not seen here).

Applied Surface Anatomy

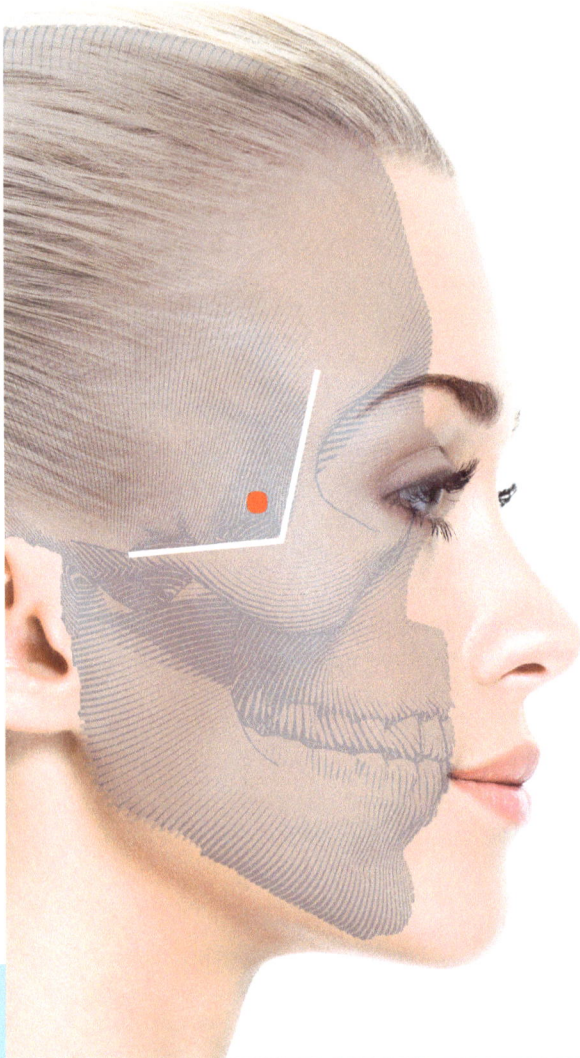

Figure 13: Surface landmarks for performing a pterygopalatine ganglion block.

Supra-Zygomatic Approach to the Pterygopalatine Block

The zygomatic arch is palpated on the side of the face (Fig. 13). This is a horizontal bony structure on the level of the inferior orbital brim. At almost 90 degrees to it, we can palpate the frontal process of the zygoma or the posterior orbital rim. Needle entry is in the corner formed by these two lines (red dot).

Applied Microanatomy of the Pterygopalatine Ganglion
Highlighting the Pterygopalatine-Trigeminovascular System (PPTVS)

This section is basically a summary of the original article by M. C. Rusu MD, PhD of the Department of Anatomy and Embryology of the University of Medicine and Pharmacy, Bucharest, Romania.[15]

In a microanatomic dissection study, the researcher set out to define as positive or negative the presence of a pterygopalatine trigemino-vascular system. He micro-dissected 18 pterygo-palatine fossae (PPF) of 9 cadaver specimens with 4.5x magnification. The content of the PPF was embedded in a consistent pterygopalatine adipose body that continued superior into the orbital apex and extended further as, what he named, a 'parasellar adipose body,' which is inferior and distinctive from the 'orbital adipose body.' Distally to the foramen rotundum, the maxillary nerve contributes fibers directly to an arterial plexus and its anterior trigeminal branches. It also contributed to the trigeminal-autonomic plexus located in the upper lateral quadrant of the pterygopalatine 'cross,' underneath the roof of the fossa. These are anastomotic branches between the PPG and the trigeminal ganglion.

The study convincingly provided evidence of the existence of an anatomically defined pterygopalatine-trigeminovascular system (Fig. 1). This would explain why pterygopalatine ganglion block would block the parasympathetic nerves to the cerebral, pia mater and dura mater vasculature and reverse the effects of noxious vasodilatation as evident in trigeminal autonomic cephalgias. The anastomoses involving autonomic and trigeminal fibers, located in the PPF passage to the orbital apex, support the complexand polymorphous neural input to the orbit, while the evidence of a pterygopalatine-trigeminovascular 'scaffold' offers a substrate for a better understanding of various facial pain syndromes.

Techniques

There are a number of approaches to performing the PPG block:

1. Supra-zygomatic approach by fluoroscopic guidance,
2. Supra-zygomatic approach by landmarks only, and
3. Suprazygomatic approach with ultrasound guidance.

4. Another option is Infra-zygomatic approach, usually with fluoroscopic guidance.
5. Finally, there's a Trans-nasal approach.

We will discuss the trans-nasal, suprazygomatic by landmarks only, and suprazygomatic with ultrasound guidance here.

Trans-nasal Pterygopalatine Block

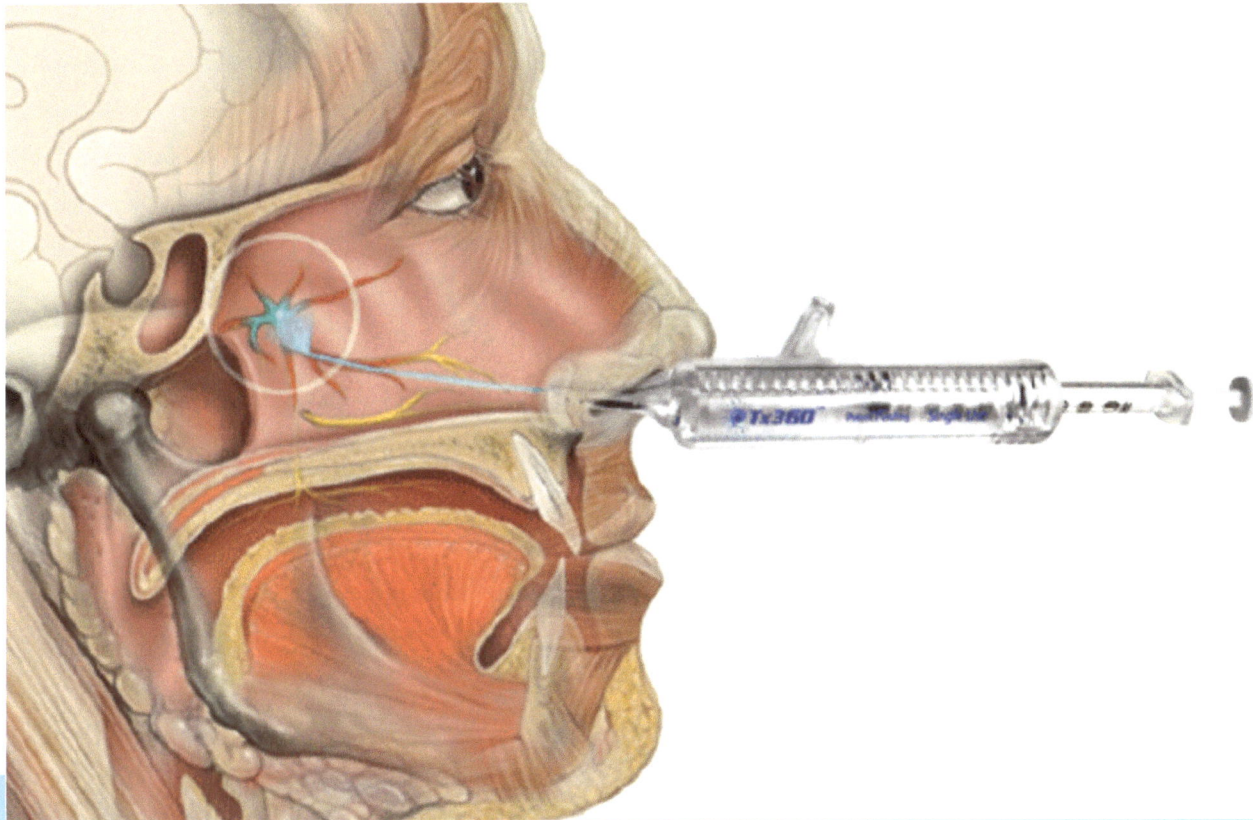

Figure 14: The Tx360 device

The Barre method is described here.[37] This method is probably as good as any of the trans-nasal approaches. It has also been described whereby a long cotton-tipped applicator was saturated with 2% viscous lidocaine and inserted into each naris until properly seated in the posterior nasophar-ynx. These were left in place for 10 minutes, then removed and resaturated with 2% viscous lidocaine before being placed in the same position for 20 more minutes,[38] and with a special apparatus designed for this procedure - the Tx360®device [39] shown in Fig. 14 (Tian Medical, Grayslake, IL, USA)

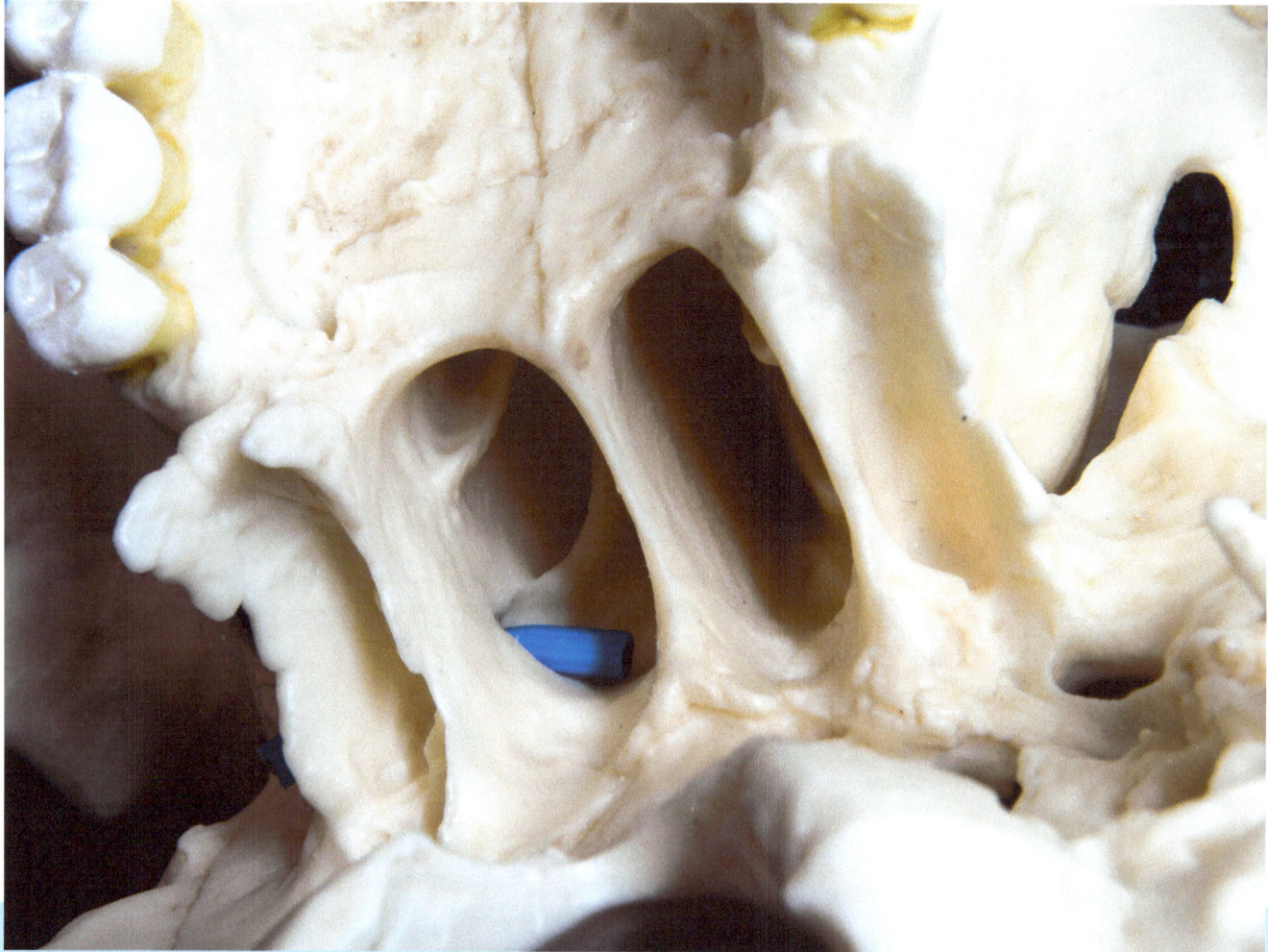

Figure 15a: A 45 degree ventral view of the bony nasopharynx. The blue marker indicates the nasal side of the sphenopalatine foramen in the posterior aspect of the lateral wall of the nose.

For the Barre method, which the patient can perform themselves on an ambulatory basis if trained properly, the patient is asked to lie supine, with their head dangling from the edge of the bed. The patient's head is then turned 30 degrees toward the side of the headache, and one puff of lignocaine 10% is squirted into the ipsilateral naris in this position (1 puff is approximately 10mg). The patient is asked to hold this position for 30 seconds. If the headache is bilateral, the application can be performed in the other nostril after turning the head 30 degrees to that side, and again holding that position for 30 seconds.

The local anesthetic reaches the pterygopalatine ganglion by diffusing through the nasal mucosa and the sphenopalatine foramen (Fig. 15a & 15b).

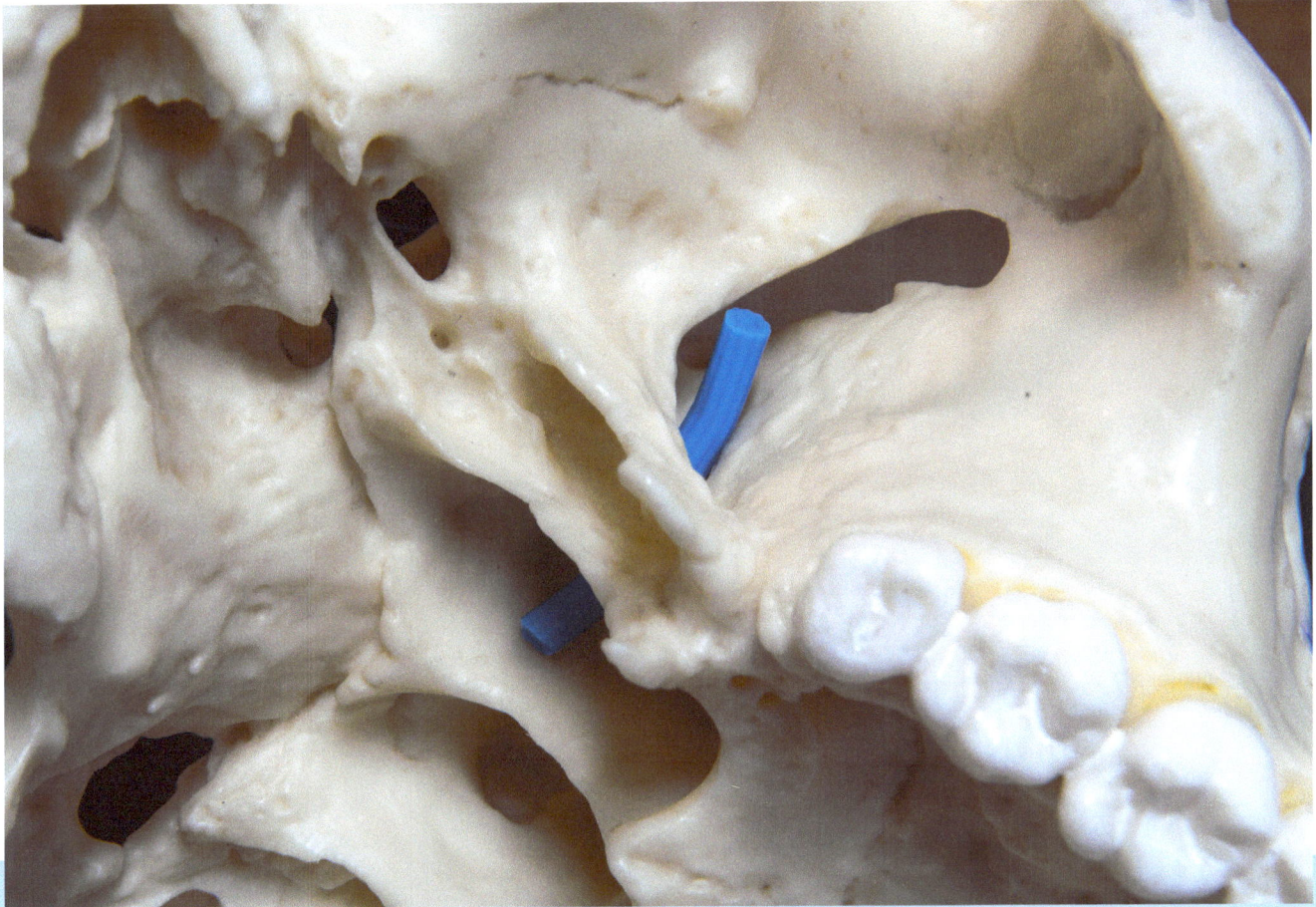

Figure 15b: A postero-ventral view of the nasopharynx, pterygoid plates and posterior maxilla: The blue marker indicates the exit of the sphenopalatine foramen into the pterygopalatine fossa.

Red line illustrates the
Frontozygomatic angle

1   Zygomatic bone
2   Zygomatic arch
3   Position of needle entry
4   Sphenoid bone

ADULT

Red line illustrates the
Frontozygomatic angle

1   Zygomatic bone
2   Zygomatic arch
3   Position of needle entry
4   Sphenoid bone

32

INFANT

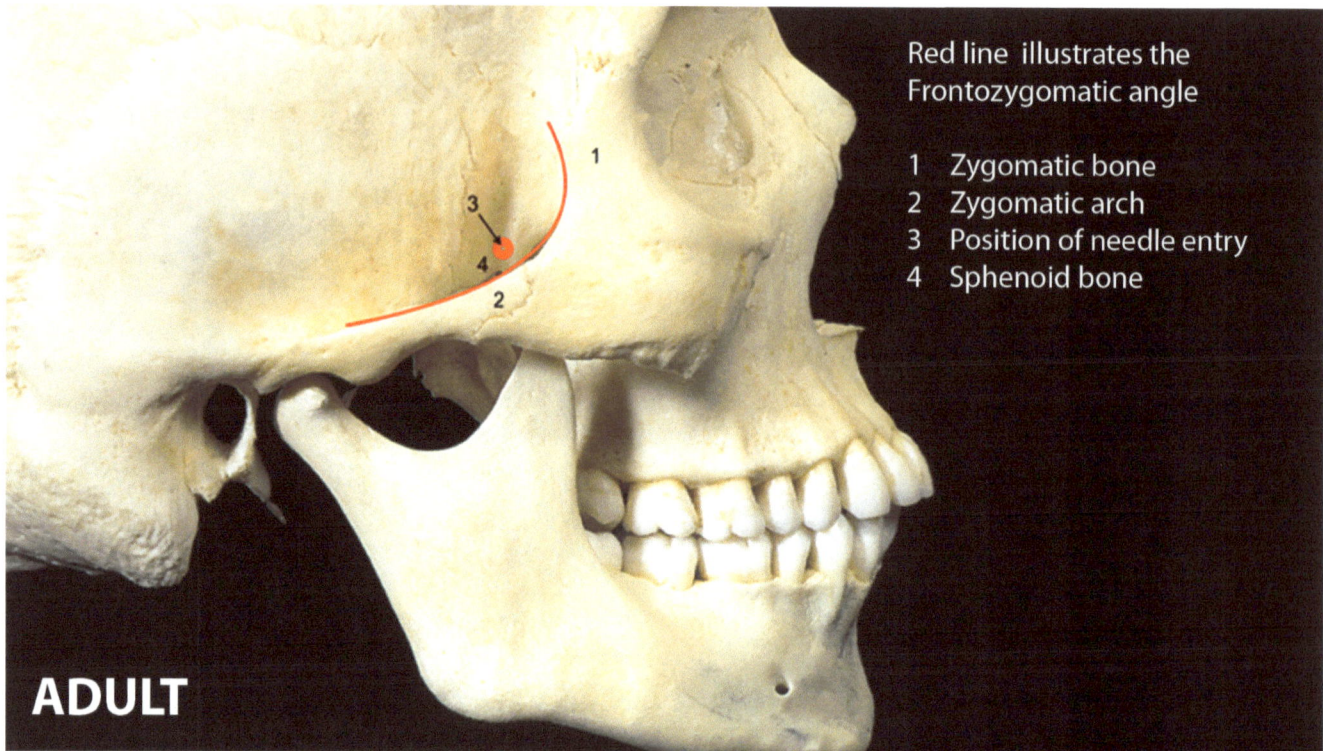

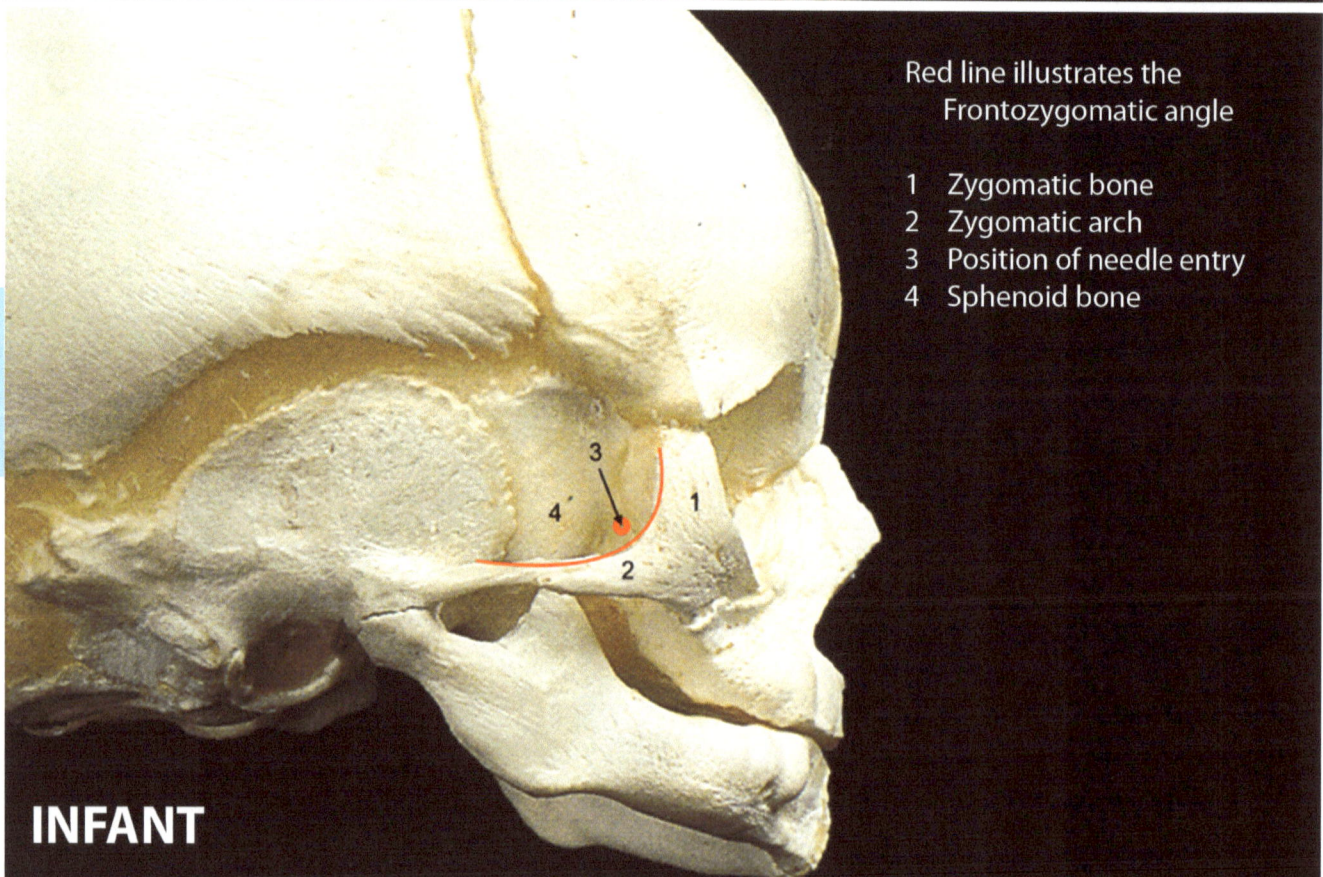

Figure 16 (top): The osteology of the right side of the face of an adult: Non-ultrasound guided landmark only technique. Red dot = Position of needle entry perpendicular to the skin Figure 17 (bottom): The osteology of the right side of the face of a baby: Non-ultrasound guided landmark only technique in babies and young children.

Suprazygomatic Pterygopalatine Block by Landmarks Only

With the patient in the supine position and the head turned slightly away from the operator, a 23 - 25 gauge 50 mm needle enters perpendicular to the skin at the frontozygomatic angle, at the junction of the upper edge of the zygomatic arch and the frontal process of the zygoma (Fig. 16).

It is then advanced to reach the greater wing of sphenoid at approximately a depth of 20 mm, then withdrawn a few millimeters and redirected 10 - 20º caudally 10º downward.

The progression in the pterygopalatine fossa is approximately 35 to 45 mm in children, and the sphenoid bone may be cartilaginous (Fig. 17). In babies and young children, it is not necessary to redirect the needle more caudad.

Loss of resistance after passing through the temporalis muscle may assist in determining the puncture depth. The pterygopalatine fossa (4) is shown in Figure 18 after the temporalis muscle (1) and zygoma (2) had been removed.

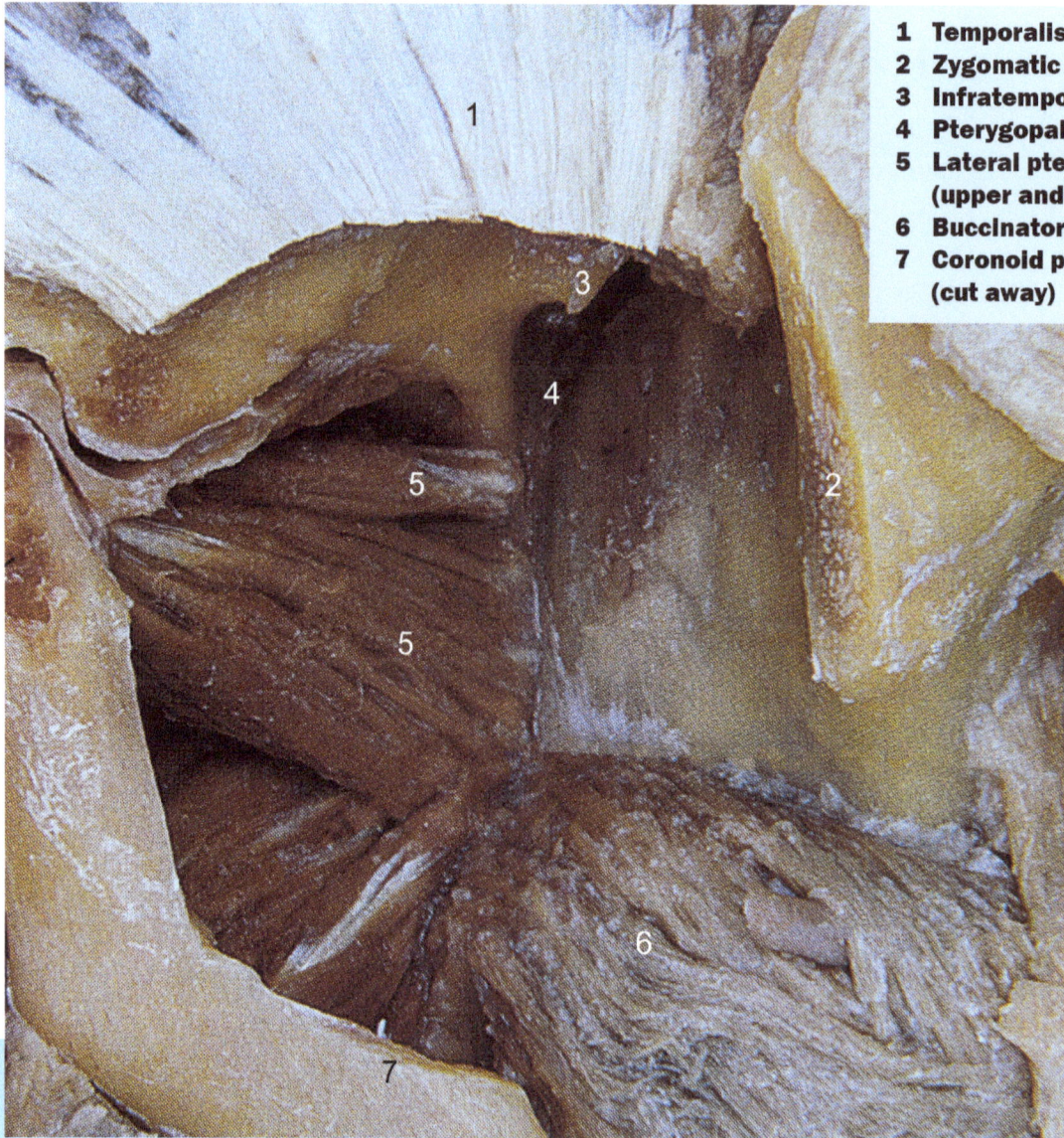

1 Temporalis muscle (cut)
2 Zygomatic arch (cut)
3 Infratemporal crest
4 Pterygopalatine fossa
5 Lateral pterygoid muscle
  (upper and lower head)
6 Buccinator muscle
7 Coronoid process of mandible
  (cut away)

Figure 18: Anatomy of the pterygopalatine fossa after removal of temporalis muscle and zygoma.

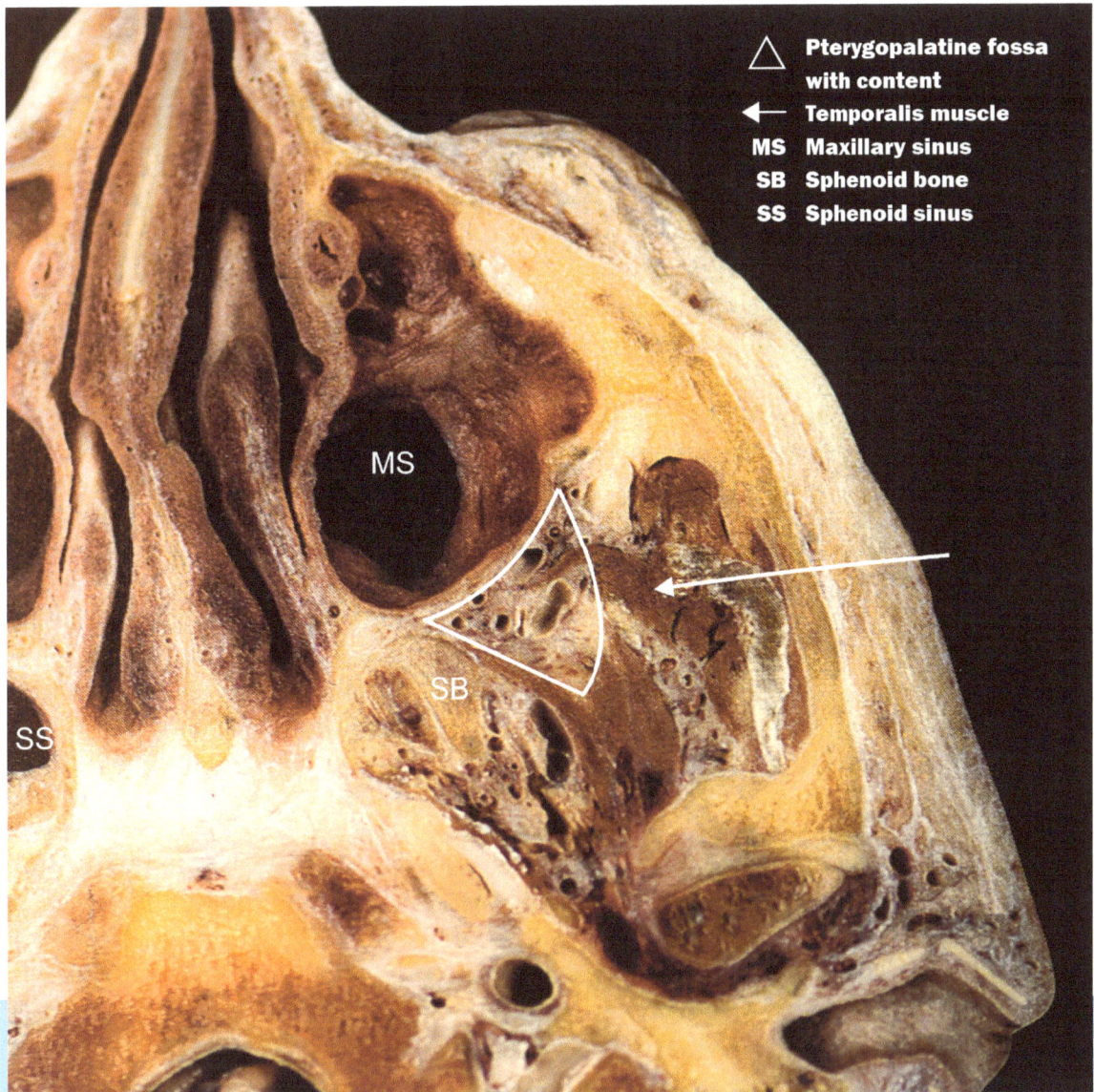

Figure 19: *Coronal section through the face showing approach to pterygopalatine fossa.*

This trans section (Fig. 19) shows the pterygopalatine fossa (triangular space) immediately deep to the temporalis muscle (arrow).

Ultrasound-guided Suprazygomatic Pterygo-palatine Block

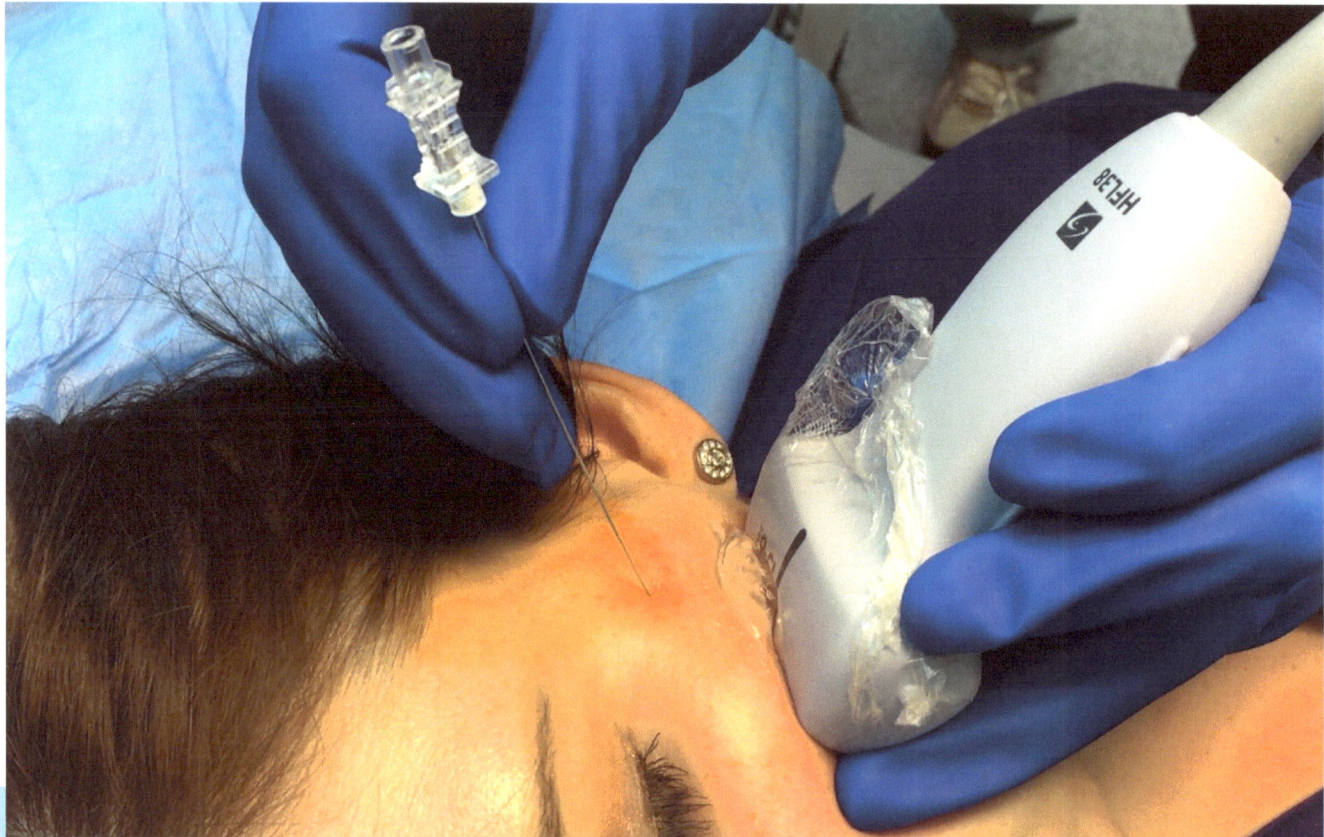

Figure 20: A 23-guage needle, open to ambient pressure, enters the skin in the corner made by the frontozygomatic angle.

Ultrasound-guidance seems to be popular as preferred technique of this block in most institutions where ultrasound is available.

A 23 - 25-gauge 50-mm needle is used. The needle puncture is again located at the angle formed by the superior edge of the zygomatic arch below and the posterior orbital rim forward (Figs. 17 & 18). The needle is then inserted perpendicular to the skin and advanced to reach the greater wing of the sphenoid at a depth of approximately 20 mm. (Fig. 20)

At this point, the needle is reoriented and advanced 35– 45 mm toward the pterygopalatine fossa. The direction of the needle and the expected mean depth of the needle tip is usually independent of the age of the patient (Refer to Fig. 16 & 17).

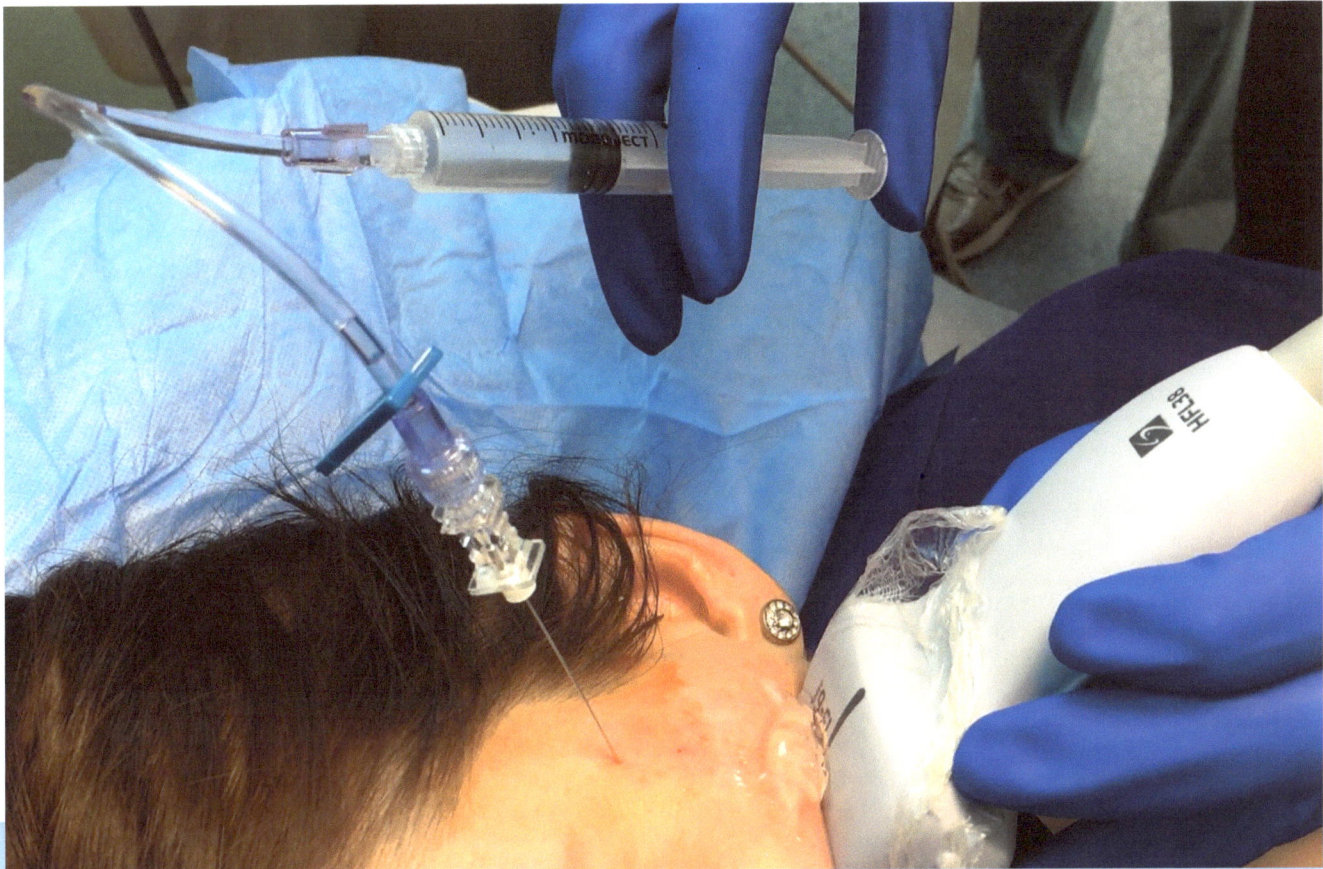

Figure 21: Local anesthetic agent is injected while observing the spread with ultrasound in the pterygopalatine fossa.

Ultrasound images are obtained with an 8–13 MHz linear array probe. The ultrasound transducer is located in the infrazygomatic area, over the maxilla (Fig. 21). The probe location allows visualization of pterygopalatine fossa, limited anteriorly by the maxilla and posteriorly by the greater wing of the sphenoid.

The needle is advanced using the out-of-plane approach, and the needle tip can usually be identified during advancement (Fig. 12). After leaving the needle hub open to ambient pressure for 15 seconds (Fig. 20), 0.15 ml/Kg of 0.2% ropivacaine is injected over 20 seconds, while observing the spread of the LA (Fig. 21) with or without added steroids. The block is usually performed bilaterally.

We recommend 0.2% ropivacaine at 0.15mg/Kg with a maximum of 5 mL for children weighing less than 34 Kg, and 5 mL (ml) of 0.5% ropivacaine for patients weighing more than 34 Kg. Steroids may be added where indicated.

References

1. Sokolov AY, Murzina AA, Osipchuck AV, et al. Cholinergic mechanisms of headaches. Neurochemical Journal 2017; 11: 194-212.

2. Cornelissen P, van Kleef M, Mekhail N, et al. Evidence-based interventional pain medicine according to clinical diagnosis. 3. Persistent idiopathic facial pain. Pain Pract 2009; 9: 443-448.

3. Ahamed SH, Jones NS. What is Sluder's neuralgia? J LaryngolOtol 2003; 117: 437-443.

4. Bowsher D. Trigeminal neuralgia: an anatomically oriented review. Clin Anat 1997; 10: 409-415

5. Peterson JN, Schames J, Shames M, et al. Sphenopalatine ganglions block: a safe and easy method for the management of orofacial pain. Cranio 1995; 13: 177-181.

6. Berger JJ, Pyles ST, Saga-Rumley SA. Does topical anesthesia of the sphenopalatine ganglion with cocaine or lidocaine relieve low back pain? Anesth Analg 1986; 65: 700-702.

7. Lebovits AH, Alfred H, Lefkowitz M. Sphenopalatine ganglion block: clinical use in the pain management clinic. Clin J Pain 1990: 6: 131-136.

8. Ferrante M, Kaufman A, Dunbar S, et al. Sphenopalatine ganglion block for the treatment of myofascial pain of the head, neck and shoulders. Reg Anesth Pain Med 1998; 1: 30-36.

9. Ruskin SL. Contributions to the study of the sphenopalatine ganglion. Laryngoscope 1925; 35: 87-108.

10. Janzen VD, Scudds R. Sphenopalatine block in the treatment of pain in fibromyalgia and myofascial pain syndrome. Laryngoscope 1997; 107: 1420-1422.

11. Saade E, Paige GB. Patient-administered sphenopalatine ganglion block. Reg Anesth 1996; 21: 68-70.

12. Piagkou M, Demesticha T, Troupis T, et al. The pterygopalatine ganglion and its role in various pain syndromes: from anatomy to clinical practice. Pain Pract 2012; 5: 399-412.

13. Seissere S, Vitti M, De Sousa LG, et al. Anatomic variations of cranial parasympathetic ganglia. Brazil Oral Res 2008; 22: 101-105.

14. Oluigbo CO, Makonnen G, Narouze S, et al. Sphenopalatine ganglion interventions: technical aspects and applications. Prog Neurol Surg 2011; 24: 171-179.

15. Rusu MC. Microanatomy of the neural scaffold of the pterygopalatine fossa in humans: trigeminovascular projections and trigeminal-autonomic plexuses. Folia Morphol 2010; 69: 84-91.

16. Bussone G, Usai S. Trigeminal autonomic cephalgias: from pathophysiology to clinical aspects. Neurol Sci 2004; 25: S74-S76.

17. Bendtsen L, Central and peripheral sensitization in tension-type headache. Current Pain and Headache Reports2003; 7: 460–465

18. Goadsby PJ, Charbit AR, Akerman AS, et al. Neurobiology of migraineNeuroscienceVolume 161, Issue 2, 30 June 2009, Pages 327-341

19. Bernstein C, Burstein R. Sensitization of the Trigeminovascular Pathway: Perspective and Implications to Migraine Pathophysiology. J Clin Neurol. 2012 Jun;8(2):89-99.

20. Schürks M, Diener H-C. Migraine, allodynia, and implications for treatment. Eur J Neurol 2008; 15: 1279-1285.

21. Yarnitky D, Goor-Aryeh I, Bajwa ZH, et al. 2003 Wolff Award: Possible Parasympathetic Contributions to Peripheral and Central Sensitization During Migraine. Headache 2003; 43:704-714.

22. Pipolo C, Bussone G, Leone M, et al. Sphenopalatine endoscopic ganglion block in cluster headache: a reevaluation of the procedure after 5 years. Neurol Sci 2010; 31: Suppl 1: 197-19.

23. Narouze S, Kapural L, Casanova J. Sphenopalatine Ganglion Radiofrequency Ablation for the Management of Chronic Cluster Headache. Headache 2009; 49:571-577.

24. Barloese M, Petersen A, Stude P, et al. Sphenopalatine ganglion stimulation for cluster headache; results of a large, open-label European study. J Headache Pain 2018; 19: 2-8.

25. Bratbak DF, Nordgard S, Stovner LJ, et al. Pilot study of sphenopalatine injection of onabotulinumtoxinA for the treatment of intractable chronic migraine. Cephalgia 2017; 37:356-364.

26. Ramachandram R, Lam C, Yaksh TL. Botulinum toxin in migraine: Role of transport in trigemino-somatic and trigemino-vascular afferents. Neurobiol Dis 2015; 79: 111-122

27. Pietrobon D, Moskowitz MA. Pathophysiology of Migraine. Ann Rev Physiol 2013; 75: 365-391.

28. Rami Burstein,Moshe Jakubowski. Unitary hypothesis for multiple triggers of the pain and strain of migraine. Neurology 2005; 493: 9-14.

29. Lamber GA, Zagami AS. The Mode of Action of Migraine Triggers: A Hypothesis. Headache 2009; 49: 253-275.

30. Karl Messlinger. Migraine: where and how does the pain originate? Exp Brain Res 2009; 196: 179-193.

31. Goadsby PJ. Pathophysiology of migraine. Ann Indian Acad Neurol. 2012; 15(Suppl 1): S15–S22.

32. Edvinsson L, Uddman R. Neurobiology in primary headaches. Brain Res 2005; 48: 438-456.

33. Levy D. Endogenous Mechanisms Underlying the Activation and Sensitization of Meningeal Nociceptors: The Role of Immuno-Vascular Interactions and Cortical Spreading Depression.Curr Pain Headache Rep 2012;16:270-277.

34. Rizzoli P, Mullally WJ. Headache. Am J Med 2018; 131: 17-24.

35. Akerman S, Holland PR, Summ O, et al. A translational in vivo model of trigeminal autonomic cephalgias: therapeutic characterization. Brain 2012; 135: 3664-3675.

36. Boezaart AP. Effects of cerebrospinal fluid loss and epidural blood patch on cerebral blood flow in swine. Reg Anesth Pain Med 2001; 26: 401-406.

37. Avcu N, Doğan NO, Pekdemir M, et al. Intranasal Lidocaine in Acute Treatment of Migraine: A Randomized Controlled Trial, Annals of Emergency Medicine, 2017, 69, 6, 743

38. Sheffield Kent. Transnasal sphenopalatine ganglion block for the treatment of postdural puncture headache in obstetric patients. J Clin Anesthesia 2016; 34: 194-196

39. Candido KD, Massey ST, Sauer R, et al.A novel revision to the classical transnasal topical sphenopalatine ganglion block for the treatment of headache and facial pain. Pain Physician. 2013 Nov-Dec;16(6):E769-78.